The
RUNN
BUCKET

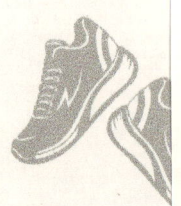

104 IDEAS TO INSPIRE
EVERY RUNNER

The
RUNNING
BUCKET LIST

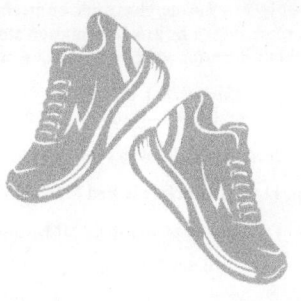

JEFF HOROWITZ

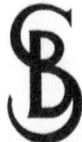

Again and forever, to Stephanie and Alex

• • •

Originally published in the United States of America in 2025 by VeloPress,
an imprint of The Stable Book Group,
32 Court Street, Suite 2109
Brooklyn, NY 11201
www.velopress.com

First published in Great Britain in 2026 by Short Books,
an imprint of Octopus Publishing Group Ltd
Carmelite House
50 Victoria Embankment
London EC4Y 0DZ
www.octopusbooks.co.uk

An Hachette UK Company
www.hachette.co.uk

The authorized representative in the EEA is Hachette Ireland,
8 Castlecourt Centre, Dublin 15, D15 XTP3, Ireland (email: info@hbgi.ie)

Copyright © Jeff Horowitz 2026
Artwork from shutterstock.com: cover and numbered list shoe © AFstudio87;
page 24 © GreenSkyStudio; page 37 © Tribalium; page 57 © Lio putra; page 68
© John Langton; page 99 © the8monkey; page 113 © SKart74; page 131 © dutko_vika;
page 157 © Blackvich; page 171 © Foxys Graphic; page 187 © Nadiiya; page 200
© KingVector; page 209 © shin28; page 214 © Kristina Bilous;
page 231 © A788OS; page 246 © Alena Divina

All rights reserved. No part of this work may be reproduced or utilized
in any form or by any means, electronic or mechanical, including
photocopying, recording or by any information storage and retrieval
system, without the prior written permission of the publisher.

ISBN 978-1-80419-381-5
eISBN 978-1-80419-382-2

A CIP catalogue record for this book is available from the British Library.

Typeset in Crimson 11.02/14.7pt by Six Red Marbles UK, Thetford, Norfolk.

Printed and bound in Great Britain.

1 3 5 7 9 10 8 6 4 2

This FSC® label means that materials used for the product have been responsibly sourced.

Please Note: This book is independently authored and published. No endorsement
or sponsorship by or affiliation with movies, celebrities, products, or other copyright
and trademark holders is claimed or suggested. All references in this book to copyrighted
or trademarked characters and other elements of movies and products are for the
purpose of commentary, criticism, analysis, and literary discussion only.
This book has been written and published strictly for informational purposes, and in
no way should be used as a substitute for consultation with health care professionals.
You should not consider educational material herein to be the practice of medicine or
to replace consultation with a physician or other medical practitioner. The author and
publisher are providing you with information in this work so that you can have the
knowledge and can choose, at your own risk, to act on that knowledge. The author and
publisher also urge all readers to be aware of their health status and to consult health
care professionals before beginning any health program.

Contents

Introduction..1

CHAPTER 1
13 Training Tips You Need to Try..........................8

CHAPTER 2
6 of the Best Ways to Build a Support Team 41

CHAPTER 3
7 Gear Choices You Need to Try 58

CHAPTER 4
13 Races Not to Be Missed 73

CHAPTER 5
8 Epic Marathons You Need to Do 93

CHAPTER 6
7 Runs in the Footsteps of Giants.......................111

CHAPTER 7
7 Ultra-Marathons, Stage Races, and Relays
You Need to Try...127

CHAPTER 8
10 Oddball Race Ideas **149**

CHAPTER 9
6 Race Collections You Need to Have **166**

CHAPTER 10
8 Ways to Give Back **181**

CHAPTER 11
4 Ways to Be a Racing Fan **203**

CHAPTER 12
9 Great Runs You Need to Experience **212**

CHAPTER 13
6 Ways to Be Entertained as a Runner **234**

CHAPTER 14
Moving Forward **257**

Acknowledgments **259**

About the Author **261**

Introduction

The term *bucket list* seems to have been around forever, and somehow, we all seem to know what it means, although few of us can remember where we first heard it or how we learned what it meant. If you told me that it originated in the Middle Ages, I'd believe you.

In fact, a specific person made up the term at a specific time not so long ago. It was 1999, and the screenwriter Justin Zackham wrote, "Justin's List of Things to Do before I Kick the Bucket." He later shortened this to "Justin's Bucket List."

The first item on Justin's list was having one of his screenplays produced. Ironically, it was years before it occurred to him that he could fulfill this wish by writing a film about a bucket list, which in 2007 became a buddy comedy film of the same name, starring Jack Nicholson and Morgan Freeman. From there it was just a short step from Hollywood to linguistic immortality.

The term may be new, but the idea existed long before the phrase was invented, although it appeared under different names. Crediting the term with the idea is like pushing on a rope; you'd have it backwards. Goals, hopes, and dreams have existed as long as humanity itself.

So, what is it about the idea of a bucket list in particular that has now captured our imagination? Perhaps it's because it gives structure to our dreams, distilling them into something defined and ordered. But it's more than just that. A bucket list is not just a string of written wishes; it's a list of goals. And as self-help author

Napoleon Hill wrote, "A goal is a dream with a deadline."[1] We're not supposed to just load items onto a bucket list. We're supposed to act on them.

Runners are especially well suited to create bucket lists. After all, most runners are constantly adding races to their to-do list: their favorite local races or their wish list of big races. Long-distance running provides hours and hours to mull this over, and the euphoria of a particularly good training day could raise our ambition—at least momentarily—and prod us into actually pursuing those goals. And then we share those ambitions with other runners.

This sharing is very important to the bucket list process. Contrary to the old stereotype, runners are not solitary beings. We are social animals. We text and chat before, during, and after our runs. A big topic of conversation is to share information about running, from training food, to workouts, to races. These conversations are fertilizer for our imagination, and from them our bucket lists grow and mature.

But discussing a bucket list is more than just idle chitchat. It's a commitment of some sort; it's a public declaration that this is a real goal of yours. It creates expectations among your peers and friends. It holds your feet to the fire to make good on your declaration, so you can maintain credibility in your group. It's also an invitation. Every mention of a bucket list item to your friends includes a question, whether stated out loud or not: Would you be interested in doing this with me? After all, if just one person wants to do a crazy thing, it sounds unreasonable, but if *two* people want to do it, well, then maybe it's not so crazy, and if three people want to do it, maybe it's something everyone should at least think about doing. Of course, there are limits to this kind of thinking.

---

1 www.brainyquote.com/quotes/napolean_hill_152852

Lemmings are a good example. Still, one of my favorite T-shirts bears the inscription, "That's a terrible idea! What time should I be there?"

Does this sound stressful? It can be, but that's the point. The right kind of pressure—self-imposed and challenging but reasonable—can be the spark that lights a fire within us and helps us achieve great things. Avoiding all stress in life is neither a good idea nor really possible. As Helen Keller said, "Security is mostly a superstition. It does not exist in nature, nor do the children of men as a whole experience it. Avoiding danger is not safer in the long run than outright exposure. Life is either a daring adventure, or it is nothing at all."[2]

Or as the writer Erica Jong put it more succinctly, "If you don't risk anything, you risk even more."[3]

By this point, you might be convinced of the utility of having a bucket list. But still, why a bucket list *book*? It's a fair question. After all, we all have imaginations and dreams. Why would anyone need help in creating their own list?

The answer is information. We can only aspire to things we know about. Sometimes it's a matter of failing to notice things that are hidden in plain sight. That requires a shift in perspective that can be supplied by someone else. Trying them out can make you a better runner, or make you feel more connected to the running community.

Other items on the list require knowledge of something you may know nothing about. It's axiomatic to say you can't have experiences you never knew about. Even the act of thinking about these items will open you up to looking at the world in a new

---

2 Helen Keller, *The Open Door* (Doubleday Books, 1957)
3 Erica Jong, *Fear of Flying* (Holt, Rinehart, and Winston, 1973)

way. You may develop the habit of looking for big experiences. As the saying goes, a mind, once enlarged, can't be shrunk again.

Can you rely on your friends and your running group to help create your bucket list? Absolutely, especially if they are adventurous and experienced. But still, the chances are that not only are there many items in these pages they haven't done themselves, but in all likelihood, there are many items they haven't even heard of. I've done over two-thirds of the items on this bucket list, including over 200 marathons—and at least one in every US State—and I'm very familiar with most of the rest of the list items. Let me share this knowledge and experience with you.

How to use this book: Think of this book, then, as an extended conversation with a very experienced runner who you know and trust. You've just posed the question, "What's on *your* bucket list?" In response, your friend just gave you over one hundred great ideas.

As you might expect, you will find running a marathon in these pages. That's the big item on many runners' wish list, and deservedly so. Running a marathon is a huge challenge, and completing one can be a life-changing accomplishment. If you decide to climb this particular mountain, you will have to decide which one to pick. In these pages, you'll find not just the obvious marathons, but many others that are sure to get your heart racing and set your imagination soaring.

Your race bucket list shouldn't end with a marathon, however. There are races of all distances that deserve to be on your list. Whether because of their unique location, their historical importance, or their unusual nature, they deserve your attention.

Most runners' bucket lists end when their race cards are full—but not ours. Your running life doesn't end at a race finish line, and neither should your bucket list. There are other experiences that every runner should have, from trying new gear and training techniques to being a fan and supporter of the sport.

Being hit with so many ideas at once can feel a bit overwhelming, even when they are organized into categories. Approach this list like you approach running itself—break it down and take it one step at a time.

First, flip through the book and become familiar with the categories. Read up on anything that jumps out at you immediately and demands your attention. Wake up your imagination and start to dream.

Next, plan to spend a little quality time with each category, imagining how you would actually make the different items on the list come true for you. This list is numbered, but you don't need to take things in any particular order. You can—and should—jump around on the list.

You may well have done some of the things on the list already. That's great—take a red marker and write "Done!" in the "Notes" section that follows every listing. Add some comments and thoughts about your experience.

Next, you can rule out the items that don't appeal to you. After all, a bucket list is a personal thing, and no two lists can be expected to look exactly the same. As hard as running and racing can be, it should still be fun and meaningful for you, even when it's difficult. If something on this list doesn't resonate with you, don't feel guilty for refusing to try it. I myself say no to other people's ideas all the time. Bungee jumping for example. I *could* do that. But I don't *want* to, and I never will.

Of the items that remain—and hopefully there will be many—break them down into three categories: the *Immediately Doable*, the *Can-Be-Done-Soon*, and the lifetime *Big Ticket* items.

The Immediately Doable ones can usually be done with little or no travel, often at little or modest expense. You can even work on several of these items simultaneously; this is particularly true of the training-related items.

The Can-Be-Done-Soon items usually involve scheduling, and so they can be somewhat out of your control. This is especially true of many races. If there are any deadlines involved for these items, put them on your calendar and commit to signing up for them as soon as possible.

The Big Ticket items are the toughest to do. These might require significant investment of time and money, not to mention emotional commitment, and years of planning. They will probably also require the understanding and support of your family and friends. But for all the effort, the items on this list might be the most rewarding. Their difficulty is in direct relation to the satisfaction you'll derive from accomplishing them. Their sheer audacity can be inspiring. Many of these can be life changing. For many people, these are the best kind of bucket list items. Daniel Burnham—the man mainly responsible for designing modern Chicago after the Great Fire—is said to have advised: "Make no small plans." Daniel would have been a great runner.

As you work your way through the list, continue to mark items as being completed in the "Notes" sections. Add comments about your experience; reading those notes later will remind you of what you have done, and help you relive each experience, its challenges and satisfactions. The final step is to pass this book around to your running friends. Let them have a chance to read the items themselves, and your notes as well. Maybe you'll find that your to-do list overlaps with theirs, and you can work together to check them off both your lists. Or perhaps you each have different item priorities, in which case you can play the old game of "I'll do yours with you if you do mine with me."

This book, then, is not to be thought of as a delicate flower, carefully handled and replaced upon the shelf. It should be manhandled and dog-eared, with folded corners, written in and filled with check marks, and bristling with sticky notes. It should be both a diary and a planner.

Now get out your marker, turn the page, and get started.

CHAPTER 1

13 Training Tips You Need to Try

- Become a Streaker *(page 9)*
- Know the Great Coaches *(page 12)*
- Take a Coaching Class *(page 14)*
- Try Yoga *(page 15)*
- Try Speed-Work *(page 17)*
- Try Cross-Training *(page 22)*
- Run Hills *(page 24)*
- Practice Running Downhill *(page 25)*
- Run in Bad Weather *(page 28)*
- Run at Sunrise and Sunset *(page 31)*
- Run Trails *(page 33)*
- Try Run Commuting *(page 34)*
- Try Strength Training *(page 37)*

Running is perhaps the simplest of all sports. Very little special gear is required, and what is needed costs little, in comparison with other sports, like skiing and golf. Best of all, we all can do it already. We've all learned this activity as toddlers, and the rules are, well, generally non-existent. There are no referees, umpires, or judges on the trails and streets. If there is a single running philosophy that could apply to everyone, it might very well be You Do You.

Having said that, however, it doesn't take most newbies long to realize that there is a lot of room for improvement for all runners. It used to be much harder to get good advice on training and racing, but the internet changed all that. The advent of online resources has been both a blessing and a curse for many runners; it is a great source of information on every possible running-related topic. That's the good news. The bad news is that this seemingly bottomless resource can be overwhelming. Where should you begin, and whom should you trust?

Let this chapter distill all this information for you. Here you will find training tips that every runner should try—from recommended workouts to how and why you should seek professional support. You don't need to take up every one of these bucket list items, but many, many runners who did, have come to swear by them. Give them a try and see what a difference they can make for you.

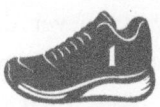

BECOME A STREAKER

In the 1970s there was a brief fad that involved people stripping naked and running through a crowded public place. Maybe it began as a dare or prank, but whatever its origin, there were soon stories of these "streakers" racing across ballpark outfields and shopping malls. There was even a pop song about it in 1974 by Ray Stevens called, yes, "The Streak."

That is *not* what we're talking about here. A *running* streaker is a person who commits to running every day, without fail. They establish their minimally acceptable workout—perhaps just one or two miles—and then they run at least that amount every day, no matter what. Feeling tired? Run. Below zero outside? Run. Getting married? Wake up early and run.

You should try being a run streaker at least once in your life. How long should your streak last? That's up to you, of course. You can decide that you will run every day from Thanksgiving through New Year's Day—39 days. Or you can commit to running every day for a year.

The longest documented running streak was established by British runner Ron Hill, who began his streak on December 20, 1964, and maintained it for 52 years and 39 days, finally ending it on January 29, 2017, at the age of 78, after feeling chest pain. During the course of his half-century streak, Hill ran at least a mile every day, despite once having a fractured sternum and, on another occasion, having to cover his mile on crutches due to a bunion surgery.[4]

If you want to make your run streak official, you can even register as a streaker on www.runeveryday.com, where you can apply for membership in the United States Running Streak Association, Inc., register your streak when it has reached at least one year in duration, and, ultimately, retire your streak. It's important here to note the fine line that exists between enthusiasm and

---

4 Jason Daley, "World's Longest Running Streak Comes to an End," *Smithsonian Magazine*, January 31, 2017, www.smithsonianmag.com/smart-news/worlds-longest-running-streak-comes-end-180961985

commitment, on one hand, and obsession, on the other. I would never recommend sticking to any running program that jeopardized your health.

For this reason, I recommend that you create guardrails before starting a streak. These should include personal rules against continuing to run when seriously injured or recovering from a serious illness, or when running would expose you to dangerous conditions, such as icy roads in sub-zero weather. It might also be a good idea to decide in advance on a stop date so that the streak does not take on a life of its own. With these limits in place, you may find that a run streak will be a great motivating tool that improves your running and reveals your unexpected toughness.

NOTES

● **BECOME A STREAKER** Date:..........................

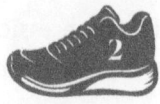

KNOW THE GREAT COACHES

Isaac Newton said, "If I have seen further than others, it is by standing on the shoulders of giants."[5] He was talking about the realm of science, of course, but his observation applies as well to the sport of running.

Running theory—how and why our bodies respond and adapt to the stimulus of running and how to maximize performance while minimizing the risk of injury—has taken over a century to develop. Every time we do a speed workout, or follow a training plan, we are benefiting from the work of coaches who came before us. To become better runners, and to fully understand our sport and our bodies, every runner should become acquainted with the great coaches and their revolutionary theories.

Start by reading books by Arthur Lydiard—*Running with Lydiard: Greatest Running Coach of All Time* or *Running to the Top* (both published by Meyer & Meyer Sport). Next, move on to Jack Daniels and read *Daniels' Running Formula* (Human Kinetics). From there you can check out Pete Pfitzinger and Scott Douglas's *Advanced Marathoning* (3rd Edition, Human Kinetics), or, for a different approach, explore Jeff Galloway's *Galloway's Book on Running: 3rd Edition* (Shelter Publications).

Exploring these giants will help you gain a better understanding of running and of your own body. Because each of us is a unique combination of genetics, motivation, and injury history, what

---

5   Maria Popova, "Standing on the Shoulders of Giants: The Story Behind Newton's Famous Metaphor for How Knowledge Progresses," *The Marginalian*, www.themarginalian.org/2016/02/16/newton-standing-on-the-shoulders-of-giants

works for one person at a given time in their lives may not work for them later, or may not work for another person. Knowing the different training approaches that have been successful over the years gives you a choice among options to see what would work best for you.

As a side note, I would recommend that you give any training program a fair chance before abandoning it for another one. I've seen runners switch programs as rapidly as a bee moves from flower to flower. In those cases, it was hard to determine what really worked and what did not. Some programs don't show results for months. Be patient, give your program a chance, and then judge the results after you complete a target race or training season.

NOTES

● **KNOW THE GREAT COACHES** Date: . . . .

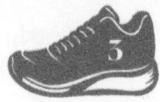

TAKE A COACHING CLASS

Reading books by coaches is great, but even better is to train to become a coach yourself. Many people do this as a stepping stone to a career in fitness, but every runner would benefit from learning the principles of coaching for their own use. By taking a coaching certification class, you will gain knowledge of physiology and biomechanics, as well as training and coaching theory. You will also be able to interact directly with your instructors, which, for my money, is a more effective way to learn than just reading a book. They can help you sift through the various training methods that you've already read about, and introduce new options as well.

By becoming a certified coach you will gain the insights you need to make informed decisions about your own training. And who knows? Maybe you could even help others to become better runners as well. You can begin by simply sharing what you've learned with your running friends, and then perhaps you can volunteer to coach a local running club. If you find that you really enjoy coaching, you can offer your services for a fee and become a professional coach.

There are many coaching programs available, both in virtual and in-person formats. England Athletics offers one of the best, and their Coach in Running Fitness (CiRF) Award is designed to prepare you to coach runners over the age of 12 to take part in non-track based activities (https://www.englandathletics.org).

NOTES

....
....
....
....
....
....
....
....
....
....
....
....
....
....

■ **TAKE A COACHING CLASS** Date:..............................

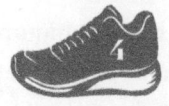

TRY YOGA

I've always avoided yoga. When friends tried to talk me into taking a class with them, I protested that I wasn't interested in any new spiritual awakening, and that time spent doing yoga could be better spent running.

I was so wrong. It turns out that the practice of yoga only includes a spiritual element if you want it to, and that the practice of yoga helps improve balance, range of motion, and core strength—all the things we need desperately to run well and injury-free. After finally trying yoga, I now practice yoga almost every day, and I wish I had started it long ago. I feel healthier and more limber, and I firmly believe it has made me a better runner.

In hindsight, I think I was actually intimidated by yoga and was worried that I would be embarrassed by my lack of flexibility and balance. I shouldn't have been concerned. Most yoga instructors and class participants are very supportive of newcomers, and everyone is too busy working on their own postures to worry about your problems. Best of all, we all get better with practice. After successfully doing a headstand for the first time, I grinned like a little kid on Christmas morning, and I couldn't wait to show off my new skill to my family and friends.

We now live in a society awash in opportunities to practice yoga. In most communities, yoga is offered at community centers, fitness centers, and dedicated yoga studios. Virtual classes are also available online, in both recorded and live formats, although that doesn't provide the personal instruction that is so helpful to a novice yogi.

When seeking out yoga classes, inquire as to the instructors' credentials and training, and when attending in-person classes, approach the instructor before class and explain that you are new to the practice. They are likely to give you special attention throughout class to help make the session productive and manageable for you. Believe me, no one is interested in seeing you fail or embarrass yourself.

NOTES

....
....
....
....
....
....
....
....
....
....
....
....
....
....
....

● TRY YOGA Date:..

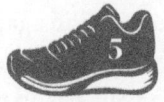

TRY SPEED-WORK

There is nothing wrong with running just for fun, with little or no structure or goals. We did that when we were kids, and we can do that now. But once we start running regularly, we notice something interesting: As we get fitter, we get faster. And that's a good thing. Running fast feels *good*. It's fun! Running fast is wired into our DNA. It's what we're supposed to do. It helped our ancestors stay alive.

At first, as we log in the miles every week, we get faster without even trying. That's because our bodies get better at delivering oxygen and fuel to our working muscles, and because our movements get more efficient. But we could only get so fast from unstructured running. At some point, we get all the possible benefit we can from that level of training. If we want to get faster, we're going to have to work for it.

That's where organized speed-work comes into play. By speed-work I am referring to a specific type of training that involves running shorter segments at fast speeds, separated by much slower, easier, recovery intervals. Coaches discovered decades ago that this format—alternating fast and slow running—triggers a physical adaptation that leads to faster distance running. It's how professionals and Olympians train for their races, and it's how you, too, can get better.

You might think that this form of training requires a stopwatch and measured distances, but that's not necessarily true. There is a form of speed-work called *fartlek*, which is Swedish for speed play. In this format, the intervals are not strictly measured; you simply pick up your pace on occasion during a run for a short period of time. Imagine you're a kid again, and you're challenging your friend to race to the lamppost. After that, you can jog easily for a while, then challenge your friend to another race to the fire hydrant. No timing or measurement is required; just run fast every now and again during your run once or twice a week.

Fartlek training will make you faster, but for the biggest improvements, you need to start timing and measuring, which usually involves finding a nearby track to run on. You might think you are not fit enough to run on a track. Not so. No one goes to the track as fit as they can be; no matter their current condition, they go there to get better. As soon as you commit to improving, you belong there as much as anyone else.

Most high schools and universities permit the wider community to use their track during non-class hours. Many community rec centers also have tracks. Standard outdoor tracks are 440 meters around, which is a quarter mile, so four laps equal a mile. Indoor tracks are generally half as large or even smaller, and the number of laps to the mile is usually posted nearby.

You can go to a track and run laps on your own, creating your own training plan, or using one that you can find online. If you run by yourself on the track, however, you would be missing one of the key elements of doing track work: making use of the energy that is generated by a group of runners. When you run with a pack, you'll likely find that you try just a bit harder than you would on your own. Perhaps you just want to keep up with the group, or perhaps you're committed to being out front this day. A good training group inspires and supports each of its members in overt and subtle ways, whether it's a high five and a compliment after a hard session, or a friendly challenge to keep up.

Finding a group to run with shouldn't be hard. Most running clubs and running stores offer regular group workouts, where a coach will call out that week's plan for everyone to follow. You may also be able to simply show up at the track and see who's there. Runners are generally friendly people, and if you see a group of runners warming up, feel free to approach them. Introduce yourself and ask them what they're working on. Chances are they'll invite you to join them.

So, what does a typical speed-work session look like? Speed workouts are measured in distances, and every athlete is tasked with running at a pace that's appropriate for them. For example, a coach may call for a workout of eight repeats of 880 meters with a 440-meter slow recovery lap between each. The pace might be set at your five-kilometer race pace. If you haven't raced and are unsure what that is, the coach may instruct you to run at a certain effort level, as measured by the *rate of perceived exertion*. That's much easier than it sounds: What the coach means is that on a scale of 1 to 10, with 10 being the absolute hardest, they may want you, in this example, to run at a 7 or 8 level.

After a while, you'll see that there are certain standard workouts that get repeated: 440m repeats, 880m repeats, 1,760m (one mile), and ladder workouts, in which you work your way up from shorter repeats to longer repeats, and then back down again, all in a single session.

Whatever your workout, expect to be tired when it's over—even as you're elated from your efforts!—and perhaps even sore or sluggish the next day. Running fast is hard work, so most coaches recommend doing it only once a week, with only a short, easy run or just rest scheduled for the next day. In fact, common practice among training plans is to have about 80 percent of all your running completed at an easy training pace. Speed-work plays only a small—though very important—role.

Does this seem too complicated? That won't last long. With regular practice, we begin to associate levels of discomfort with specific speeds, and we learn how to run by feel. It's like learning to drive a manual transmission car; after a while, you get to know when to shift by the sound of the engine, and you really begin to handle the car like an expert. Speed-work will enable you to do the same with your own body.

One of the greatest benefits of doing speed-work is that you learn precise pacing. Each interval—whether a quarter mile, half mile, or full mile—will be run at a different pace, since you can't maintain the same top speed at a longer distance as you can over a shorter one. After a while, you can begin to associate a given pace with an effort level. That's the key that opens the door to having control over your running, because if you can sense your pace, you can make pacing decisions and become a truly purposeful runner. You can follow a race plan, and you can take calculated risks about deviating from it, because you will be in complete control of your running.[6]

And, of course, there's just that speed thing. You will undoubtedly get faster, and as we've said before, running fast is fun, especially on race day.

NOTES

---

[6] Of course, you can also do your speed-work running on a treadmill instead of on a track. Many of us prefer running outdoors, and if you run on a treadmill you won't get the benefit of running with other people, but treadmill running provides precise speeds and a safe and comfortable environment. The physiological benefit of treadmill running versus outdoor running has stirred up a lot of debate, but the difference is really negligible, so go with whatever works best for you.

● TRY SPEED-WORK Date: ....

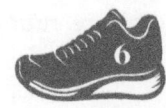

TRY CROSS-TRAINING

Runners like to run, of course. Most of us don't run so that we can do other things—we run to run. But if all we do is run, we often leave ourselves open to injury. Whether it's from underused muscles or accumulated stress from pounding the streets, it seems that sometimes running takes from us as much as it gives.

Give your body a break from this routine once or twice a week by switching to another endurance training mode. Whether it's indoors on a cardio machine, like an elliptical trainer or spin bike, or outdoors, on a road bike or on inline skates, or by doing strenuous trail hiking, do something to build your cardio base—your "engine," in coaching jargon—while giving your joints a rest. You're not cheating on your running; you're saving it. Commit to giving it a try.

Are all cross-training options created equal? Not really. The elliptical trainer comes closest to mimicking the running motion, while indoor spinning or outdoor cycling helps improve running—and prevent injury—by strengthening those muscles that running typically doesn't work: the quadriceps. Swimming is great for injury recovery and building cardio fitness, but it is less likely to directly improve your running. Rowing might be the best to build your VO2 max—that is, the volume of oxygen that you can absorb in a given amount of time, which is a key measurement of cardio fitness.

So what's the best option for you? Simple: The one that you like the most is the one that you'll probably keep doing. Or rotate between them to keep things from getting too routine and boring, and to build better overall fitness.

NOTES

● **TRY CROSS-TRAINING** Date: ....

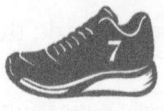

RUN HILLS

It's an old saying among coaches—"Hills pay the bills." You may never love them. You may never even like them. But they get the job done. They build your running strength and improve your running form—after all, no one can over-stride when running uphill, and you naturally will swing your arms more forcefully as you push uphill.

Hills have also been called speed-work in a disguise, since the power that you develop on the hills will help you run faster. Many runners begin their training season with a few weeks on the hills before they move onto the track, or they alternate weekly speed-work with hill-work.

There is no one true way to run hills. You can find a 200-meter steady incline and run up and down repeatedly for a strenuous workout, or you can incorporate hills into your regular running route in a less formal fashion. If you don't have any hills nearby, you can run repeats on a ramp in a parking garage—though keep an eye open for cars!

Whatever you decide to do, aim to include hills in your running at least once per week. You'll notice the difference it makes in your strength, speed, form, and confidence.

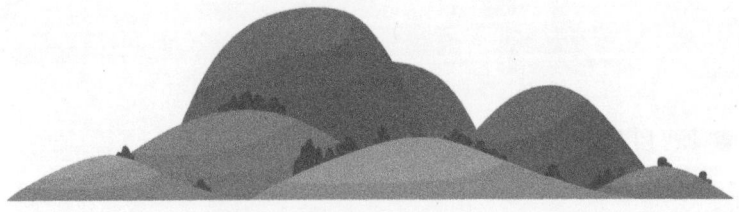

NOTES

....
....
....
....
....
....
....
....
....
....
....
....
....
....
....

● **RUN HILLS** Date: ....

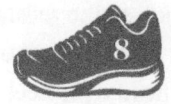

PRACTICE RUNNING DOWNHILL

Running uphill is hard. If you took the preceding recommendation to heart and gave it a shot, you know that by now. But once you're at the top of a hill, the only way to go is down. How you do that will make the difference between being a good runner and a great runner.

Think of running uphill as being like putting money in the bank. When you reach the top, you're rich. If you run downhill slowly, it's like just throwing all that hard-earned money away. But if you can manage to run downhill fearlessly, you'll spend that money in the best way possible, by running fast with little effort. Put downhill run training as something that you should add to your bucket list.

You can add downhill running to your training regimen the same way you can add uphill running and speed-work: in a measured format, doing repeats, or in a less formal way, by adding some downhill running to your regular runs. But if you are doing uphill repeats already, keep your downhill running for another day; if you try running hard both uphill and downhill, you won't last long. The point of interval training, you might recall from our section on speed-work, is to alternate hard and easy segments.

You might think that running fast downhill would be easy, but that's not necessarily the case. It can be scary. You may feel like you're on a roller coaster without a seatbelt, and that you're about to lose control and tumble. And you might. But with practice, you can learn to control your descent while running fast. Think of downhill running as being like a controlled fall. The key is to maintain a *high leg turnover*, that is, to have a high number of total steps per minute. Every foot-strike reestablishes contact with the ground and will slow you down just enough to maintain control and keep you from going head over heels.

An important part of this is to maintain a slight forward lean. When you lean back, you are putting on the brakes. That's why we do it, after all. Fight that urge, keep your feet moving, and fly down that hill.

Begin your downhill sessions by choosing an easy to moderate downhill stretch to run, and increase your speed just slightly until you feel comfortable and secure. Then, over time, try to pick up your speed bit by bit. When this feels good, try running down a slightly steeper hill.

Don't rush your progress. If you feel unsteady and likely to fall, slow things down. Then get back at it. If you continue to practice these repeats, you'll develop the confidence to blaze downhill in training, and, more importantly, in racing.

NOTES

● **PRACTICE RUNNING DOWNHILL** Date:..........................

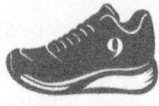

RUN IN BAD WEATHER

As a coach, I tell my athletes there are beautiful days—and there are running days.

While we may enjoy a warm, sunny day, the ideal weather for running is chilly with overcast skies, perhaps even with a bit of drizzle. While we may not feel comfortable when we walk out the door, we are sure to feel better after a few miles of running, when our internal furnace has warmed us up.

Some of my most memorable runs, however, did not take place in these relatively mild conditions. Rather, they involved notoriously bad weather, the kind that makes most people want to stay in bed under the covers. I certainly do not advise you to ever go outside in dangerous conditions, like during a lightning storm, but if the weather is safe but just uncomfortable, then lace up your shoes and head out the door. You may experience the run of a lifetime. You will certainly increase your confidence to be able to handle whatever Mother Nature might throw at you on race day.

TORRENTIAL RAIN. Remember: It's only water, and once you're soaked to the bone, you can't get wetter. Wear a cap to keep at least some of the rain out of your eyes, and wear lightweight shoes that won't feel like cement when they get wet. But remember, also, that water draws heat from the body quickly, especially when it's chilly outside, so wear something warm, and get out of your wet clothes and into something dry as soon as possible when you're done.

Here's a tip on running through puddles: When you see one, pick up your pace and run hard through the puddle. Your harder foot-strike will displace water, and your speed will get you out of there before the water splashes back on your foot. Of course, use your discretion if you're running with other people: They might not appreciate being splashed by you.

SNOW. Running in a snowstorm can be a beautiful experience, especially if there is no wind. Equally memorable is running right after snow has fallen, before sidewalks are shoveled and streets are plowed. Wear trail shoes, or, even better, wear running cleats over your shoes.[7] Don't worry about the mileage; running in snow can wear you out quickly, so just get out for a short but glorious run, at whatever speed you can maintain, and then get back home for a cup of hot chocolate. You'll have earned it.

A side note: Always be wary of black ice when running in winter. I've taken more than one bad spill on ice that I never saw. Protect yourself from falling by keeping your run stride short where the footing is suspect. That will keep your center of gravity almost directly over your feet, which will help you recover quickly if your foot slides on a patch of ice.

STORMS. This is not an option that is available to everyone, and it's one that requires great discretion, but a run in a storm is a once-in-a-lifetime kind of experience. I live in Washington, D.C., where we are occasionally the end stop for hurricanes. By the time one reaches my doorstep, it has lost much of its power. But like a bear in a cage, it's still a wild animal and needs to be treated with respect. When I've headed out the door on those occasions, I was exhilarated by the gusts of wind I encountered, and felt like I was in a real adventure.

---

7 Yaktrax, for example, is one brand of running cleats you may consider using.

If you decide to run in high winds, make sure you are not putting yourself at an unreasonable risk—there are some conditions that you should never run in!—and keep the run short. Avoid any downed power lines, and be wary of debris.

On one such run in a weakened hurricane about 20 years ago, my plan was to follow my usual route by crossing a bridge over the Potomac River. When I got to the bridge, I wisely decided to stay on my side of the river, and headed home. At that point I came up with a rule that I've shared with all of my runners and clients, and which I apply to all aspects of my life: Be smarter than you are brave. There are times when you can do something, but you should not do it.

A bit of final advice: It's a good idea to always let someone know when and where you go for a run, especially if you head out alone (read about runner IDs on pages 33 and 71), but this is even more important if you head out in bad weather.

NOTES

....

....

....

....

■ **RUN IN BAD WEATHER** Date:..

RUN AT SUNRISE AND SUNSET

If running in bad weather is like being on a roller coaster, then running in the early morning and early evening is like meditating to classical music. At those times you can experience a sky more lovely than the most beautiful painting that you've ever seen. Combined with the natural repetitiveness of running and your steady, rhythmic breathing, it's not hard to slip into a state of quiet awareness, an almost meditative bliss.

It's moments like these which make me not only happy that I'm a runner, but happy to be alive. If I'm struggling with something or otherwise feel bad, I will inevitably feel better, and if I'm feeling ok, I'll end up feeling on top of the world.

Like the best meals, these moments can be shared with friends, creating memories that you can both look back on years later, especially if it takes place at an exotic location during a vacation. Or you can keep these runs to yourself, carving out a moment that is reserved for you alone to enjoy. Of course, just as with running in bad weather, please put your safety first and do not put yourself in any potentially dangerous situations.

NOTES

....
....
....
....
....
....
....
....
....
....
....
....
....
....
....

● **RUN AT SUNRISE AND SUNSET** Date: ....

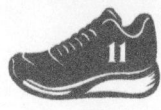

RUN TRAILS

Some runners never let their shoes wander off asphalt, and that's a mistake. Running on trails will improve fitness because varied terrain forces the body to make micro adjustments on landing, and these little changes add up to a different training stimulus than taking the same steps over and over again on a flat surface.

Running trails also forces us to pay attention to every step, since daydreaming trail runners may soon find themselves face down in the dirt. This heightened engagement, where every step has to be considered, can be more interesting and engaging than running on streets; every step is a puzzle to be solved.

But we don't run trails just because they make us more fit; we run them because of the beauty that we find out there. Whether you are lucky enough to live near a national park, along a river or in the mountains, or anywhere there is some green space to enjoy, heading out on a trail gives us a chance to see how uplifting a run can truly be.

A few words again about safety: Just as with running in bad weather, please let someone know where you're going if you plan to run alone on a trail, or better yet, run with someone else. Be aware of any reports of wild animals in the area, or the possibility for a sudden storm. I recommend you make sure to bring an ID, a cell phone, and even a small basic first-aid kit, containing an elastic bandage, some adhesive bandages, a few alcohol prep pads, and some antibiotic ointment.

NOTES

....
....
....
....
....
....
....
....
....
....
....
....
....
....
....
....

● **RUN TRAILS** Date:...

TRY RUN COMMUTING

Training and racing are a big part of every runner's life, but it all usually occupies a space that is separate from the rest of their days. For most runners, running is a refuge from all the stresses of living, and a place where they can lose themselves. But for most of us, it's also a completely isolated part of our lives. If running and the rest of your life were friends of yours, it's a safe bet you have never introduced them to each other.

All of that is fine, but every runner should try to break through the wall that separates their running from the rest of their lives, to achieve something like a seamless lifestyle.

The easiest way to do this is to figure out how to use running as a practical way to get around. As a thought experiment, imagine if it would be possible to run part or all of your daily commute to work or school. Are there any errands you could do while running, like a trip to the post office or to the grocery store for a few items? How about casual events, like meeting up with a friend for coffee? Could you run to those?

Incorporating running into your daily life like this is not without challenges. You may have to buy some specialized gear, like a running backpack or waist pack. If you live too far away from some of your destinations, you may need to brainstorm possible ways to do at least some of the route on foot by using public transportation only part of the way, or parking midway between your home and your destination. You may need to run only one way and use a car or public transportation for the return trip. You may also need to figure out how to handle a possible need to change clothing. All of these challenges can be difficult, but there are usually solutions.

Once you go through the trouble of overcoming the challenges, you'll find there are many benefits to merging your life this way. By driving less, you will save money and reduce your contribution to global warming. You will also save time, even if your errands and commuting take longer, because you won't have to carve out more time during the day for your workouts.

You might be wondering how all of these short runs could possibly be as effective as a single long run. It might surprise you to hear that many of the benefits that you get from a single long run will also result from doing several shorter runs during the course of a day. That's because the stress you put on your body by running is cumulative; it's as if you pick up where you left off with your run. And, of course, you don't have to completely eliminate your single long runs. For most of us, that's what the weekends are for.

Finally, the best reason to work running into your daily life is that it delivers the same basic benefit as your long run does: It usually leaves you happier than when you started. And isn't that a great thing to get more of during your day?

NOTES

● TRY RUN COMMUTING Date:.....................................

TRY STRENGTH TRAINING

Cross-training will help you build your endurance base, but strength training will help you build strength in specific skeletal muscles, making you more fit overall, and reducing your risk of injury.

Most runners seem to think that lifting weights or working on strength machines will make them too big. That fear is unfounded. First of all, even if it is your goal to get big, it's hard work and requires a singular focus to achieve. It's unlikely to happen with a moderate program, and it certainly won't happen by accident. Second, there are many types of strength-training programs, each with a different focus and goal. I suggest that you choose one that will be in support of your running.

Another misconception about strength training is that it will take too much of your spare time, leaving you with less time to run.

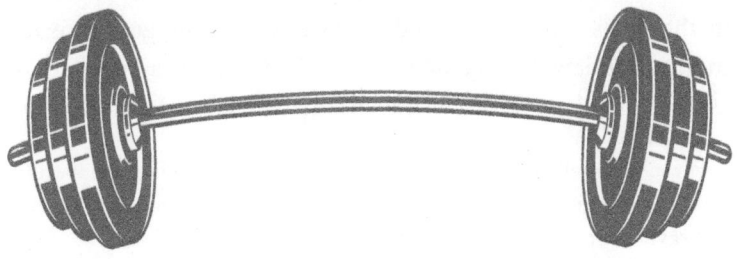

That's generally untrue. Yes, you will have to devote some time to your weekly strength workouts, but this likely will take far less time than you imagine. Even a little bit of strength work creates measurable improvements. Two or three workouts a week of just 20–30 minutes on non-consecutive days can do the trick. Weigh that against the time you would have to spend away from running if you are injured, and it sounds like a reasonable investment.

Once you commit to adding strength training to your workout routine, you need to decide what you need to do. A lot can be discussed in this area, but here are the basics of what you need to know: Work on improving your core strength, and focus on functional strength training.[8]

You can join a fitness facility and hire a personal trainer, or find one to meet you in your home. Some trainers even offer outdoor group sessions, often in a boot-camp format. You can have a trainer help you with every workout, or set you up with a routine and then meet with you periodically to update it, or simply get you started with a few sessions and send you on your way. There is no single right approach.

You may also benefit from joining group classes. Whether focused on training with small dumbbells, or core-centered format classes like Pilates, these classes could be more affordable and fun than working with a trainer or on your own.

If you decide to work with a personal trainer, I recommend that, at a minimum, you schedule at least three sessions to start. In those sessions you should explore what your goals are for training, review the overall program, learn and practice a set of exercises, and agree on several specific workouts to do on your

---

[8] For more detailed information on this topic, as well as advice on specific exercises and workouts to perform, see my book *Quick Strength for Runners: 8 Weeks to a Better Runner's Body* (VeloPress).

own. Most of my own clients opt to continue to meet regularly after these introductory sessions so I can monitor their practice and keep their workouts challenging and productive.

Your choice will depend entirely on whichever format you feel is most comfortable, is most affordable, and works best for you. Some self-honesty here goes a long way. If you are not self-motivated in the gym, or feel lost when you're there, maybe you need to schedule more sessions with a trainer. But if you feel you know, basically, what to do and why you are doing it, and feel comfortable working from earlier instructions, you might be fine on your own.

Whatever you choose, remember that a little bit of expert instruction up front is an insurance policy against getting hurt later on your own. Invest in yourself. As the hair coloring advertisement used to say, because you're worth it.

Still unconvinced? Remember: Some 90 percent of all chronic running injuries are caused by weakness or imbalance in the core muscles—that is, the abdominal and gluteal muscles of our midbody—front, sides, and back—which act as a foundation for all movement. If those muscles are weak, then our running mechanics get compromised, excessive stress is placed on certain muscles, tendons, and ligaments, and presto! We suddenly experience pain somewhere, and have to lay off running for a time.

A good strength-training program can prevent that. Focus on a mode of training that builds core strength, such as Pilates classes, and aim to do complex movements that engage a large number of muscle groups. Not only will this make your workouts more efficient, but they will also make them functional, making you more prepared for the tasks of regular life, including running. Looking better on the beach is just an added bonus.

NOTES

● TRY STRENGTH TRAINING Date:.............................

CHAPTER 2

6 of the Best Ways to Build a Support Team

- ☐ Join a Running Club *(page 42)*
- ☐ Try a Running Camp *(page 44)*
- ☐ Hire a Coach *(page 47)*
- ☐ Hire a Massage Therapist *(page 49)*
- ☐ Hire a Dietitian *(page 53)*
- ☐ Get a Gait Analysis *(page 55)*

An old African saying, which has now become part of our popular culture, is that it takes a village to raise a child. I would add that, similarly, it takes a team to create a strong, healthy runner. It may be possible to be a runner without having a support group, but why not give it a try? I'm betting you'll find you are a better runner for it. Whether it is a group of like-minded runners, or professional trainers and healthcare providers, having a group of people to keep you on track—literally—can be worth its weight in golden running shoes.

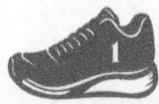

JOIN A RUNNING CLUB

There's a myth that runners are solitary creatures who prefer to run alone. The more than 56,000 runners who competed together in the 2025 London Marathon would beg to differ. Humans are social beings, and in this regard, runners are no different from everyone else. Most runners find that they enjoy running in a pack instead of running alone. If you never have, you should give it a try.

Running with a group can be as easy as finding some friends who agree to meet regularly for a little trot. It can also involve showing up for regular group runs organized by the local running shop. Either one will provide you with an incentive for getting out of bed and out the door, if only because there are people who are expecting you to show up, and who might razz you if you miss a training day.

If you are planning to register for a race in your upcoming running season, you may be able to coordinate your race preparation with your new running friends. Your local shop may also offer fee-based seasonal training programs, from a beginner's "Couch to 5K" class to a coached marathon-training program. But for the maximum number of opportunities and level of support, I recommend that every runner, at least once in their running lives, join an organized running club.

The experience of belonging to a running club can vary according to the size of the club. Your local running club may have a few dozen members and a staff of part-time volunteers or it may be a far larger affair. But what all run clubs have in common is that they provide a place for committed runners to train and race together on a regular basis.

Most clubs organize long runs and track sessions regularly, and many arrange for discounts in local running stores and races. Most importantly, they provide a place for like-minded people to come together, which often leads to lasting friendships.

To find a running club near you, check with your local running store, or search for your local group via England Athletics or the Strava app.

NOTES

● JOIN A RUNNING CLUB Date: ....

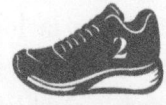

TRY A RUNNING CAMP

If you're reading this book, you're probably interested in becoming a better runner and having memorable running experiences. For most of us, this means fitting in training—and reading about training—wherever there's free time in our schedules. Usually work, family, and social commitments compete for our attention. Perhaps you've daydreamed, as many of us have, what it would be like to be a full-time professional runner. You would have all the time in the world to focus on becoming the best runner you could be.

You may never reach that pinnacle of running, but you could do the next best thing: Attend a running camp. These are like organized running vacations, ranging from four to seven days, held at beautiful locations across the UK, Europe, and even the US.

Running camps typically offer more than just an opportunity to meet other runners and explore stunning guide-led training runs—although they do include those. They typically also offer informational seminars and related services, from nutrition and training classes to fitness testing.

These camps are essentially like resorts in that they offer the opportunity to reenergize yourself, body, mind, and soul. Think of them less as an extravagance, and more as an investment in yourself. You'll reap the dividends for years to come.

Camps can vary quite a bit in cost and services offered. Among the ones you can look into are:

WOMEN ONLY RUN RETREATS. Locations worldwide, with a variety of outdoor experiences offered. (Website: www.runwildretreats.com)

WILD RUNNING. Offer UK-based retreats in stunning locations such as the Lake District and Dartmoor. The emphasis is on connecting to the landscape and nature. (Website: https://www.wildrunning.co.uk/)

RUNNING TRIPS. Offer training camps in the UK and Kenya for various levels. (Website: https://www.runningtrips.co.uk/)

ZAP ENDURANCE RUNNING VACATIONS. An all-inclusive camp for goal-oriented runners, offering personalized coaching and lectures on training theory, programs, and nutrition, in a resort located in the mountains of Blowing Rock, North Carolina. (Website: www.zapendurance.com/running-vacations)

RUN WILD RETREATS. For women only, these retreats are designed to help women find joy in running, away from expectations or the pressures of daily life.

NOTES

....
....
....
....
....
....
....
....
....
....
....
....
....
....

■ **TRY A RUNNING CAMP** Date:......................................

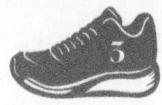

HIRE A COACH

There's a common misperception among many runners that only elite athletes hire professional coaches. That's simply not the case. In fact, all runners can improve by working with a certified professional coach, and inexperienced beginner runners in particular might benefit the most.

Running is an unusual sport in that almost all of us assume we already know how to run when we begin. After all, most of us have been running since we were just a few years old. A novice golfer or swimmer would likely have no problem signing up for lessons with a pro, knowing they will need help mastering the essential skills, but hiring a run coach would never occur to most runners.

That's a mistake. Few of us understand the biomechanics of running, and how to use that knowledge to run more effectively. Further, training principles are often not intuitive and are not generally taught in school. Every runner should experience what it's like to have a coach design a program customized just for them, with their specific history and goals in mind.

Perhaps you've educated yourself on running theory and technique, and perhaps you've even taken a coaching class yourself, all of which was suggested in Chapter One. There is still great value in having another expert help shape your training and racing program.

In the field of law (my first career, before fitness), there is a saying: An attorney who represents himself has a fool for a client. Often, this is true in running as well. We may find it hard to view our program—and any injuries—objectively.

I've handled this myself by wondering what I would tell myself at different times if I were a client of mine. I've been surprised that the answer sometimes was very different than what I was actually considering beforehand. While this approach was helpful, it was still flawed in that I was limiting myself to my own imagination, even if it were redirected. A better approach would have been to get a second opinion. Every runner should try relying on a coach's expertise and experience to shape their program.

Finding a coach is easier than you might think. You can start by asking around among your running friends. Your local running store will also likely be able to offer referrals, and some of the employees there may be coaches themselves. A local running club might be able to recommend coaches as well.

Organizations such as England Athletics and Bark.com have details of running coaches across the country on their websites.

Wherever you find your coach, make sure to ask about their credentials, training, experience, and coaching philosophy. The best coaching relationships are based on trust, and that comes from openness and an ability to communicate effectively. Interview your prospective coach to get a sense of what it would be like to work with them, and remember: Trust and communication go both ways. To get the most from your coaching experience, you will need to be clear about your training and injury history, your goals, your availability, and your level of commitment.

NOTES

....

....

● HIRE A COACH Date:...

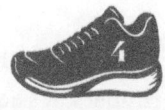

HIRE A MASSAGE THERAPIST

Runners pound their bodies. That's the truth of running. While we hope to avoid injury, that's often just a price that we have to pay to do the thing we love.

Still, there are ways that we can reduce the risk of injury, speed healing, and treat ourselves better. Regular massage does all of this and should be at the top of any list of runners' self-care treatments. If you haven't tried it yet, you should.

Regular massage helps move waste products from our muscles, break up the adhesions that form between damaged muscle cells, and release tension in stressed muscles. The result of this is quicker recovery from hard runs, better range of motion, and fewer aches and pains.

For many people, the image of a massage involves gentle rubbing and relaxation. That is true in some forms of the practice, like Swedish massage. That's not what we're talking about here. Therapeutic, deep-tissue massage can be uncomfortable and even painful, as the massage therapist works to manipulate the muscle and break up those adhesions. I've been on the verge of tears during many a massage. But the more frequently you get a massage, the more supple your muscles will be, and the less discomfort you are likely to experience during the session.

If we compare massage therapy to dental care, we can easily see how this works. If you don't get regular cleanings, your eventual visit to your dentist can result in painful dental work to eliminate the decay that's occurred. But if you practice good dental hygiene, including regularly scheduled cleaning visits, you'll likely have a much easier time.

With this in mind, you can now see that getting a therapeutic massage isn't a luxury for runners; it's actually a great investment in your health, and it's worth every penny.

So how often should you schedule your visits? I've never heard there's ever been a problem with someone getting *too many* massages. I would get one every day if I had the time and money. But realistically, you should aim to get a massage every month, or even better, every few weeks, especially if you are working through an injury or physical problem and have got a big race coming up.

Over time, regular massage will help keep you on the roads and out of the doctor's office. I credit weekly massage with helping me overcome a hamstring problem and enabling me to complete the Comrades Marathon, an ultra-marathon run in South Africa (more on that race later).

Once you commit to massage, you will need to decide how to work it into your race schedule. You wouldn't want to get a deep-tissue massage right before your race because you want to feel fresh on race day, and a deep-tissue massage can sometimes leave you a bit sore.

You also might not want to get deep-tissue massage right after a race either. A race creates more damage to your body than you would experience in training, as you push yourself harder than you do in training. You can witness the proof of this the day after a major marathon, as runners limp their way across city streets, or through the airport concourse on their way home. Those runners have created micro-tears in their muscles, and those will need time to heal. A deep-tissue massage would only cause more damage and slow the healing process.

If you are going to get a massage right before or right after a big race, you should only get a gentle massage, with the goal of aiding blood flow and relaxing the muscle. The time for therapeutic massage will come later.

Now that you're convinced, you need to find a massage therapist. That shouldn't be hard. Your friends—especially the athletes you know—might have some practitioners to recommend, and you can get referrals from your healthcare provider or doctor. You can also ask about referrals at your local health club, spa, or chiropractor. If there is a massage school near you, that could be a good place to inquire as well. An online source to look into is the SMA (The Sports Massage Association) (website: http://thesma.org).

Finally, a quick word about professionalism. Massage practitioners are part of the healthcare delivery system. They are trained to provide care in compliance with industry standards and codes of conduct to ensure that you feel safe and secure as they provide their services. Before you book any sessions, check references and ask the therapist about their background and credentials, as well as about how the session will proceed. You may also ask about pricing, and whether they offer package discounts.

NOTES

● HIRE A MESSAGE THERAPIST Date: . . . .

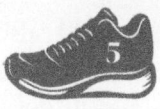

HIRE A DIETITIAN

Hiring a dietitian is much like hiring a coach or a massage therapist, in that it's often enlightening and beneficial for us to get expert advice on something we generally take for granted or think we already know all that we need to know.

As runners we make more demands on our body than most people, and that requires us to pay more attention to how we fuel ourselves. Not knowing how to eat properly as an athlete is like having a high-performance race car but not knowing what kind of fuel it takes.

Runners need more carbohydrates than most people to power workouts, and more protein to facilitate recovery. In addition, we need proper amounts of electrolytes to maintain proper muscle function, and vitamins and fat to ensure healthy hormone production and cellular function. A good, healthy, balanced diet would take care of all of this, but how many of us feel confident that we are eating everything we need and avoiding the things that hurt us?

A good dietitian can give us guidance on these things, and also measure our metabolism to determine our actual—not theoretical—calorie needs. They can also draw up a detailed eating plan for you if you want one. All of this can be very enlightening and should be experienced by every runner at least once in their lifetime.

Finding a good dietitian should not be that hard. You can go the usual route and ask for referrals from running friends, employees at running stores and fitness centers, and your healthcare provider. You could also look online through the Health & Care Professions Council (HCPC) (website: https://www.hcpc-uk.org/check-the-register/) for a practitioner near you.

Understanding the relevant terminology and credentials could take a little work but is an important step. First, you need to understand the difference between a dietitian and a nutritionist. Simply put, a dietitian has undergone the required education and certification; a nutritionist may have also received a similar education, but not necessarily, because the term "nutritionist" is not licensed. Every dietitian, therefore, is a nutritionist, but not every nutritionist is a dietitian.

Similarly, the rest of your support team might know a few things about nutrition, but unless they are licensed dietitians, they should not be giving you detailed nutritional guidance and advice. You can use your personal trainer to help you with strength training, and your coach to help design your running program, but do not rely on them to structure an eating plan. In technical terms, nutrition is beyond the scope of their practice. When interviewing potential experts, be sure to ask about their credentials. You should also ask about their area of expertise; some practitioners specialize in sports nutrition and can help you fine-tune your nutrition for peak performance in training and racing.

NOTES

....
....
....
....

....
....
....
....
....
....
....
....
....
....
....

● **HIRE A DIETITIAN** Date:...

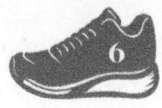

GET A GAIT ANALYSIS

Not all runners move the same way. Some look smooth as silk, and others look like they're doing their impression of a building falling down. We all seem to know intuitively how proper running should look—we know good running form when we see it—but few of us could explain why someone who seems to be running poorly is doing what they are doing.

All of this can be explained by a physical therapist practitioner or exercise physiologist. When proper running form is compromised, there are specific explanations for what is going on. And each deviation from proper form brings a higher risk that at some point an injury may occur.

You may know this already. Perhaps you've had a running injury, and you've gone to physical therapy and learned what you are doing wrong, and how to fix it. If so, I hope your problem has been solved and you are back out on the roads. Still, for you, and also for everyone who hasn't yet worked with a physical therapist, it would be a good idea to get your overall running form critiqued by a trained professional.

A gait analysis involves having you run on a treadmill while a practitioner films you and then analyzes your form in slow motion. A gait analysis can reveal if there is an incorrect running pattern, which can be traced to an underpowered muscle group that isn't doing its job, or tightness somewhere that is limiting proper range of motion. Getting this done before you get injured can help you avoid a world of problems down the road, and help you improve your performance right now.

You may be able to get a salesperson in your local running store to put you on a treadmill for an analysis, but they are likely not fully trained in what to look for, and can't match the level of expertise that a physiotherapist brings to the table. Make the investment and schedule a gait analysis at a physiotherapy clinic. It will be worth it.

NOTES

....
....
....
....
....

⦁ **GET A GAIT ANALYSIS** Date: ....

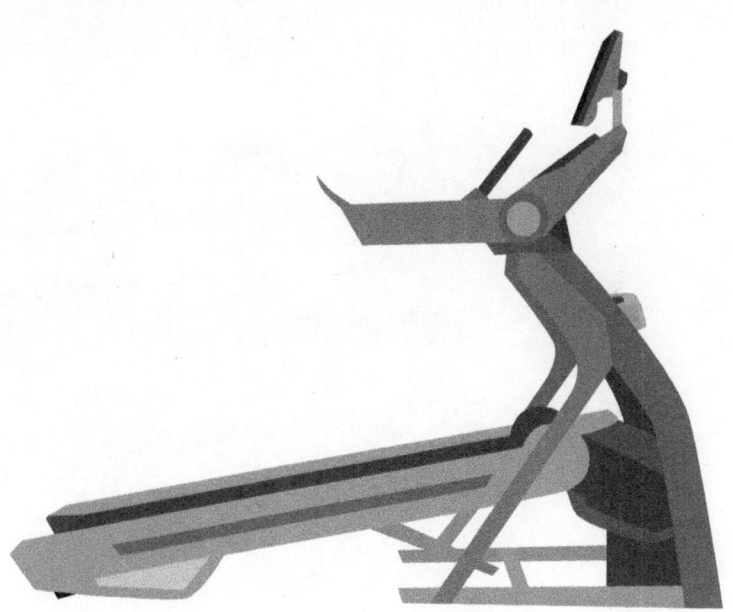

CHAPTER 3

7 Gear Choices You Need to Try

- ☐ Use a Training Log *(page 60)*
- ☐ Use Recovery Tools *(page 62)*
- ☐ Try a Pair of "Super Shoes" *(page 64)*
- ☐ Try Hi-Tech Clothing *(page 66)*
- ☐ Get a Good Running Watch *(page 68)*
- ☐ Run with No Devices *(page 69)*
- ☐ Run with ID, Money, and Your Cell Phone *(page 71)*

Runners don't require a lot of stuff. We don't need to buy balls, rackets, or clubs. We need special clothing and shoes, but nothing as specialized as skis and softball or baseball mitts, and what we buy to run in can later be worn to go to the gym or just walk around. That's one of the truly great aspects of running: The price of entry is as low as you need it to be.

Beyond the essentials, however, there is some gear that all runners should try at least once in their lifetime. You may find that some of the equipment listed next doesn't do much for you, and that's fine. Running still comes down to putting one foot in front of the other the old-fashioned way.

I love running as much now as I did when I went for my first training run, wearing an old shirt, ratty shorts, and a pair of tennis shoes. But that outfit is long gone, replaced by much more comfortable and functional clothing that makes my running even more enjoyable.

Make use of the gear that works for you, and which makes a difference in your running life. But you were a runner before you had all this, and you will still be a runner without them. Don't believe any marketing campaign that tells you anything different.

Still, you might find that some of these items are game changing for you. Either way, give them a chance and form your own opinion. Or, as I will suggest on page 69, try running without any of it at all.

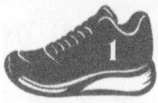

USE A TRAINING LOG

Beginner runners go for jogs, often on a random schedule. There's nothing wrong with that. But experienced runners usually have a plan, especially if they are training for a race. They work to improve their endurance and speed, with a specific target date in mind for a big challenge, whether it's a local race, a major international marathon, or the Olympic Games.

What many of these athletes have in common is that they track their workouts in a training or racing log to create a database of their performance. This enables them to later judge their preparation and the effectiveness of their workouts. Did they overtrain, get injured, or fail to reach their target peak? The training log will tell all.

You should try this approach at least once in your life. You can log your workouts in an online site or app, create your own using a spreadsheet, or go old-school and use a pad or pages in a binder.

What should you include? The general answer is: as much information as possible. Include performance data, such as your workout mileage, time and pace, route, and any elevation or hills on the course. Include information about your gear, such as the clothing and shoes you wore. Note the weather conditions. Add in how you slept the night before, and what you ate and drank before, during, and after your workout.

More subjectively, critique your run—did you feel like you were floating on air or running through wet cement? How was your frame of mind? Happy, sad, annoyed? Were you preoccupied with anything? The more you write, the more data points you will have later to judge why a training plan did or did not work for you, and why you did or did not get injured.

Keeping a written record of your training not only will serve as a valuable diagnostic tool, it will help you document important moments in your life. Special days will be memorialized for you to recall later, like the day you saw an eagle soaring during a run, the sound of your footsteps on freshly fallen snow, or your thoughts about other events in your life as you ran. It will serve as a diary of the major accomplishments in your life, helping you to recall how you prepared for your first race, or the most challenging race of your life. For these reasons, it's not uncommon for athletes to save their logs after each season and create libraries of them.

NOTES

● USE A TRAINING LOG Date: ....

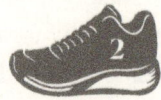

USE RECOVERY TOOLS

Think of your body as a race car. It performs wonderfully, but without proper maintenance in the shop, it can't perform on the roads. For runners, this means using available tools to keep muscles pliable and healthy, to minimize the impact of running, and to speed recovery. We've already talked about how every runner should try therapeutic massage, but there are many tools available for runners to use to care for themselves on a daily basis; tools that are cheaper and more time-efficient than scheduling daily massage sessions.

At the top of your list should be a foam roller. Originally a tool available just in physiotherapy clinics, foam rollers are now widely available in an impressive array of sizes and shapes. Whether they are soft or hard, full length or travel size, smooth or knobbed, or even vibrating, all foam rollers provide a form of *self-myofascial release.* That's a fancy term for self-massage of your connective tissue. While this might be uncomfortable, regular foam rolling will give you many of the benefits of regular massage.

Similarly, an electric massage gun can help massage sore muscles and speed recovery. I like to use it on all soft-tissue areas I can reach; not just my quads, hamstrings, and calves, but also my lower back, shoulders, and even the soles of my feet and my palms. There are many brands available, ranging widely in price. Check the power and speed of each to determine which is the right model for you; in the long run, an underpowered massage gun may not be worth the money you've saved.[9]

Finally, consider investing in electronic sequential massage sleeves. These are sleeves that zipper up your legs from your feet to your hips and inflate in a variety of available patterns, to varying degrees of intensity, depending on how you program them.

Think of one as a big blood pressure cuff that you can pump up, squeezing your legs from the bottom up. It was originally developed for people with circulation problems, but companies soon realized that endurance athletes could benefit from using this machine after long, grueling workouts and races. Is this an essential tool? Maybe not. But every runner should at least try it and decide for themselves. If you go to the expo for a big race, you will likely see vendors offering demonstrations, which is a cost-free way to give this a go.[10]

NOTES

. . . .

. . . .

. . . .

. . . .

---

9 One product that has worked well for me is Hypervolt (website: www.hyperice.com).

10 Two brands that are worth taking a look at are Air Relax (website: www.air-relax.com) and Normatec by Hyperice (website: www.hyperice.com).

● USE RECOVERY TOOLS Date:

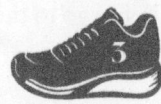

TRY A PAIR OF "SUPER SHOES"

Nike was the first company to come out with a revolutionary kind of running shoe that featured a carbon fiber plate in the forefoot. Named Zoom Vaporflys, these shoes arrived in 2017 and were designed to change the way the foot moved on impact and push-off. Soon, world records began to drop, and other shoe companies began to sell their own versions of these "super shoes."

To understand how these new shoes work, it helps to understand just a little about how our feet work. The human foot serves two opposing purposes while running: to provide a soft and responsive base to land on, and then to provide a stiff platform from which to push off.

In accomplishing these two tasks, some compromises are made. Because our feet need to be supple on landing, they cannot be entirely rigid on push-off, which means some energy is lost. By placing a stiff carbon fiber plate in the shoe, Nike minimized the energy loss and turned the foot into a more efficient lever.

This sounds great, but there's a price to be paid for this innovation, both metaphorically and literally. By decreasing the foot's natural impact-absorbing characteristic, these shoes may put more strain on a runner's Achilles tendons and raise the risk of an injury there. For that reason, it's recommended that runners give their bodies a chance to adapt to the shoes by slowly increasing the time they spend running in them from week to week.

And the cost. Wow. Decades ago, industry analysts wondered if consumers would ever pay £100 or more for a pair of running shoes. The answer was a resounding yes. But a pair of super shoes can cost over three times that amount. Still, all considered, that might not be such a high price to run like a world champion. Treat yourself to a free test ride at your local running shop and see for yourself how they feel.

NOTES

....
....
....
....
....
....
....

● **TRY A PAIR OF "SUPER SHOES"** Date: ....

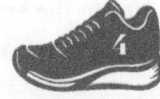

TRY HI-TECH CLOTHING

When I first began running, I did what many new runners were doing at the time. I simply pulled on an old cotton T-shirt, threw on a pair of cotton shorts, slipped on my old tennis shoes, and headed out the door.

How far we've all come since then. First, cotton gave way to technical clothing made of polypropylene or some other lightweight, breathable material that helped keep us cooler in the summer and warmer in the winter.

The next generation of clothing brought fabrics made of bamboo or silver thread, which made the clothing antibacterial. Gone was the old sweat-stink that survived every wash.

The newest gear innovation is smart clothing, which uses nanotechnology to weave tiny, powerful sensors into its fabric—now called e-textiles—to measure and record biometric data. First developed for first-responders, medical personnel, and the military, this technology can also make your clothing part of your coaching team.

Sounds like something from a sci-fi movie? Well, the future is now. Among the products currently available are training socks that have sensors to measure data on foot-strike, delivered to an app that can track running technique, steps, speed, altitude, and distance traveled. Also available are yoga pants that monitor whether a pose is being performed correctly. If a body part is out of alignment, sensors will vibrate, alerting the wearer that they need to adjust their body position.[11]

Will these tools be worth the price tag they carry? Will they help us perform better? I'd like to see for myself, and so should you.

NOTES

---

11 These products are Sensoria Smart Socks and Nadi X Smart Yoga Pants, respectively.

● TRY HI-TECH CLOTHING Date:..................................

GET A GOOD RUNNING WATCH

There are now so many high-tech options available for our sports watches that it's almost hard to remember when a running watch simply had a timer option.

Modern watches track speed, heart rate, your sleep, and a whole host of other biometrics while tracking your running route, taking phone calls and texts, and monitoring the weather, your altitude, and ground wind speeds. For those of us old enough to remember the Dick Tracy comic strip, where the detective was able to receive and send messages via his space-age watch, this seems truly fantastic.

For the modern runner, a good watch is an indispensable training tool. There are several brands available that track all your necessary metrics and provide, to a greater or lesser degree, a seamless interface with your phone. No longer will we need to be alone when we run, even when we are by ourselves.

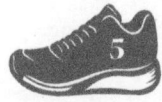

NOTES

....
....
....
....
....
....
....
....
....
....
....
....
....
....

● **GET A GOOD RUNNING WATCH** Date: ....

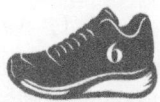

RUN WITH NO DEVICES

This might seem to be a strange bucket list item, since we just reviewed all the hi-tech gear you should be trying. Nevertheless, every runner should try training—and even racing—with no electronics at all. No tracking devices, personal music devices, watches, or phones. Nada.

The benefit of doing this is that with nothing to distract you from your running, you can be completely aware of everything that you're experiencing, which will enhance your awareness of your running.

In coaching, we call this "associative running," and it's practiced by elite runners to improve their performance. Instead of letting themselves become distracted by music or other feedback—which we call "dissociative running"—they focus on what they are doing. They monitor their breathing, their energy, their biomechanics, their effort level, and a host of other items on their mental checklist. They also focus more on the trail or road on which they're running, as well as on weather conditions. They turn running into an immersive experience and use this awareness to work with their bodies to improve their running.

The ultimate test of this associative running is to race without a watch. Using your sense of pacing, based on the knowledge of your perceived effort that you gained from your track workouts, you should be able to meet your race goals—or come pretty close—just by feel.

If you are of a certain age and a fan of certain movies, this might ring a bell. You should think of yourself as being like Luke Skywalker in his bombing run against the Death Star in the first released *Star Wars* movie, subtitled *A New Hope*. Luke disengaged his electronic guidance system and relied on his senses—the Force—to guide him to success. You should do the same.

Do I run this way myself? No, not yet. But I aim to try. It's on my bucket list.

NOTES

■ **RUN WITH NO DEVICES** Date: ....

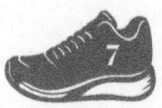

RUN WITH ID, MONEY, AND YOUR CELL PHONE

We mentioned this in our section on trail running, but safety concerns aren't just limited to when we are out in the woods on dirt trails. I was on a pre-dawn run a few years ago, running down a dark street, when I tripped on a crack in the pavement and fell. I got up, brushed myself off, and continued on my way, but I couldn't help but wonder what would have happened if I had had a bad accident. I realized I did not have any identification or money on me, nor did I have my phone. If I were somehow knocked cold and rushed to the hospital, I would have been a John Doe.

Don't put yourself in a position of being unable to get help or help yourself, and don't put your family and friends in a position of not knowing where you are. There are running tights that have side thigh pockets for cell phones, and waist belts with pockets for ID, money, and cell phones. There are also custom runner ID wristbands and ankle bracelets available that can be engraved with your personal information and emergency contacts.

NOTES

● RUN WITH ID, MONEY, AND YOUR CELL PHONE   Date:............

CHAPTER 4

13 Races Not to Be Missed

- Do a Parkrun *(page 74)*
- Run a Santa Run 5K *(page 76)*
- Run The London Landmarks Half Marathon *(page 77)*
- Run a Valentine's Day Race *(page 78)*
- Run a Race for Life *(page 80)*
- Run Bay to Breakers *(page 81)*
- Run the Beat the Boat 10K *(page 83)*
- Run the UK's Longest Underground 10K *(page 84)*
- Run the NYRR Midnight Run *(page 86)*
- Run a Mystery Race *(page 87)*
- Run a Women's Race *(page 89)*
- Run in the Great Ethiopian Run *(page 90)*
- Run The Great North Run *(page 92)*

This is the ultimate bucket list category. For many runners, the goal of training is to run a race. Sure, training improves our physical and mental well-being, but racing is fun! It inspires us and motivates us to get out the door on those mornings when we would much rather stay in bed.

You don't have to push yourself hard to enjoy a race, although many runners do. You also don't have to travel to exotic lands to enjoy racing, although many runners do that too. In the world of road racing, there are as many different types of races as there are people who run them.

I like to think of races as flavors of ice cream in a local sweet shop. If you've somehow never had ice cream, you really need to give it a try. You can start with the basics, like vanilla, strawberry, and especially chocolate. Those can all be wonderful. But then wander down the counter and look at all the incredible options. Rum raisin! Rocky road! Who wouldn't want to try them all?

This book will be your guidebook to the sweet shop of racing. Here you will find all the best flavors, picked especially for you.

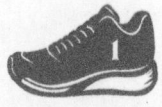

DO A PARKRUN

Parkrun is a free community-organized event where people come together to walk, jog, or run a 5km course every Saturday morning. It began in 2004 in Bushey Park in London, and has grown into a global phenomenon taking place in over 2,000 locations across 23 countries.

One of the best things about Parkrun is how inclusive it is. People of every age and fitness level are welcome and there is no time limit. If you're already a Parkrun regular, maybe try taking part in a race next time you visit a new place.

Parkrun is staffed solely by volunteers, so they're a great place to tick off more than one of your bucket list items (see Be a Race Volunteer, Thank the Volunteers and Police on a Racecourse, and Cheer!).

To find out more, visit https://www.parkrun.org.uk

NOTES

● **DO A PARKRUN** Date:..

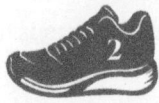

RUN A SANTA RUN 5K

Anyone can run on a beautiful spring or summer day, but sometimes it's hard to get up the enthusiasm for a winter workout. Get motivated by this event, which encourages participants to dress up in full Santa suits. Santa runs take place across the country and there is no expectation in terms of your pace or finishing time.

Most Santa runs encourage you to raise money for charity. It's quite the spectacle with some events attracting up to 3,000 Santas, all running for a good cause!

NOTES

● RUN A SANTA RUN 5K Date:..............................

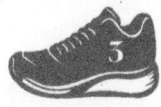

RUN THE LONDON LANDMARKS HALF MARATHON

If you like the idea of doing some sightseeing during your next run, then the London Landmarks Half Marathon could be just what you're looking for.

Billed as the only half marathon to go through both the City of London and the City of Westminster, the course takes you past some of London's most iconic sights. Taking in impressive architecture such as The Shard and the Walkie Talkie Building, runners will also trot past St Paul's Cathedral, Nelson's Column, and the Bank of England. If that isn't enough to entice you to sign up, this race encourages participants to raise money for charity, with over £70 million going to good causes so far. (Website: https://llhm.co.uk)

NOTES

....
....
....
....
....
....
....
....
....
....
....
....

● RUN THE LONDON LANDMARKS HALF MARATHON   Date: . . . .

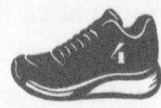

RUN A VALENTINE'S DAY RACE

The perfect date run, this February event has a fun theme that gives runners the chance to run in a costume. Be bold! This is a late-winter event that is meant to be more fun than challenging, so get out there with your sweetie and get into the spirit of it. Here are some suggested races:

THE LOVE RUN, GLASGOW. Whether you're single or already taken, the Love Run in Glasgow, Scotland, is a great way to celebrate St Valentine.

As well as a Singles Run of either 5 or 10K (perfect for meeting fellow runners looking for love), there is a Couples Relay and a Speed Dating Run, which pairs entrants with a new partner for each kilometer of a 5K. (Website: https://www.letsdothis.com/o/up-and-running-events-156202)

NOTES

■ **RUN A VALENTINE'S DAY RACE** Date: ....

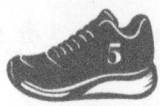

RUN A RACE FOR LIFE

Race for Life is more than a fundraising event—it's a nationwide movement powered by hope, unity, and determination. Organized by Cancer Research UK, it invites people of all ages and backgrounds to walk, jog, or run in support of life-saving cancer research. Whether you're tackling a 5K, 10K, or diving into the mud with Pretty Muddy, there's a challenge for everyone. No finish time, no pressure—just purpose.

It all began in Battersea Park, London, in June 1994. Back then, 750 women came together and raised £48,000. That spark ignited a fire. Today, Race for Life has grown into a powerful force with over 10 million participants across more than 400 locations in the UK. Together, they've raised over £970 million—funding breakthroughs like radiotherapy, which helps over 130,000 people in the UK every year.

Originally a women-only event, Race for Life evolved to reflect the spirit of inclusivity. In 2019, it opened to men, and now welcomes everyone—regardless of gender, background, or fitness level. Whether you're a seasoned runner or just starting out, you're invited to take part in something bigger than yourself.

People join for deeply personal reasons: to honor loved ones lost to cancer, to celebrate survivors, to stand in solidarity, or to challenge themselves. Every story adds to the collective heartbeat of the event. Every step taken is a step toward progress.

You don't need to be an athlete. You just need to show up. Every stride helps fund research, every moment raises awareness, and every participant brings us closer to a future free from cancer.

NOTES

....
....
....
....
....
....
....
....
....
....
....
....
....
....

● RUN A RACE FOR LIFE Date:.................................

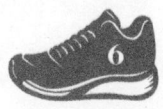

RUN BAY TO BREAKERS

Held on the third Sunday in May in San Francisco, this 12K/7.46-mile race was first run in 1912 to lift the city's spirits after the 1906 earthquake. Its name reflects the course route, which starts a few blocks from San Francisco Bay and finishes adjacent to the Pacific Ocean, where waves break on the beach.

Bay to Breakers set the world record for the largest footrace in the world in 1986 when it had 110,000 participants. The course has changed a bit over the years, but it's always been a grand tour of the city, running through Golden Gate Park, past the Conservatory of Flowers to the Great Highway.

What makes this race truly special, however, is its party atmosphere. While racing naked is no longer allowed—much to the dismay of some longtime nude runners—many participants choose to race in costumes. This is encouraged by the race itself, which has established a special race category for "centipedes" which are teams of 13 or more runners linked together by bungee cords or other "safe mechanisms."

To understand the race philosophy, look no farther than the 2025 official race slogan: "Ready to Get Weird?" (website: www.baytobreakers.com).

NOTES

● RUN BAY TO BREAKERS Date: ....

RUN THE BEAT THE BOAT 10K

A truly unique trail race is the Beat the Boat 10K race in Eton & Windsor. You'll not only be competing against other runners, but a target pace boat full of spectators that will be trying to beat you to the finish line.

Set against the backdrop of Windsor Castle, most of the race follows the Thames Path. You can choose to race against one of five boats that are traveling at different paces (40, 50, 55, 60, and 70 minutes). There's also a 1-mile fun run for children, making this a wonderful way to inspire the whole family to take part. (Website: https://www.beattheboat.com/)

NOTES

● RUN THE BEAT THE BOAT 10K Date:..............................

RUN THE UK'S LONGEST UNDERGROUND 10K

Taking place regularly in the historical city of Bath, the Two Tunnels race is a truly special running experience. The course has the longest underground section for each race distance in the UK!

The Somerset & Dorset Railway closed in the 1960s and was sealed until 2013. The first tunnel (The Devonshire Tunnel) is 408m long, while the second (Combe Down Tunnel) is 1,672m long—both are well lit and have been resurfaced for the enjoyment of runners, cyclists, and walkers.

With an ultra marathon, 50K relay, marathon, three different half marathons, two different 10Ks, 5K, 2K, and 500m Colourburst races, there are events for everyone. (Website: https://www.relishrunningraces.com/bath-two-tunnels-railway-running-races.php)

NOTES

● **RUN THE UK'S LONGEST UNDERGROUND 10K** Date: . . . .

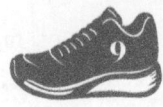

RUN THE NYRR MIDNIGHT RUN

Why pay for an overpriced evening of too much drinking and forced good cheer when you can usher in the New Year in a race? This new tradition has caught on in cities and towns across the world but perhaps the best of the lot is organized by the New York Road Runners Club—the folks who bring you the New York City Marathon.

Held in Central Park, this 4-mile race kicks off with a countdown at 11:59 p.m. Runners set off on the park's inner loop, enjoying cider at the rest stops, and ushering in the new year with apples and pretzels at the finish line. But the star attraction has always been the iconic Central Park itself, and the wonderful city it calls home. (Website: www.nyrr.org/races/nyrrmidnightrun)

NOTES

....
....
....
....

● RUN THE NYRR MIDNIGHT RUN Date:........................

RUN A MYSTERY RACE

If you are finding that your running routine is getting a little tiresome, then running a mystery race might be just what you need to pep you up.

The Drop organizes races where participants are picked up by a bus, then blindfolded and taken to a mystery location to be dropped off. The challenge is to make it back to headquarters with no tech, no map, no watch, and no idea where you are. You are given a tracker so that the organizers can keep an eye on you for safety reasons.

With events running across the UK, a mystery race is a fantastic way to find a new running route and enjoy a sense of true camaraderie with your fellow runners. (Website: https://www.thedropuk.co.uk)

NOTES

....
....

● RUN A MYSTERY RACE Date:.....................................

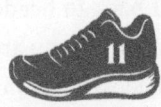

RUN A WOMEN'S RACE

This, of course, is not something that could be on everyone's bucket list, but women runners should consider adding it to theirs.

It's hard to imagine now, but there was a time when women were not allowed to run in organized races. It was thought they were too frail to push themselves in a race—especially a long-distance race—and would suffer permanent physical harm if they tried to do so.

Such nonsense has now been discredited, but for many years, participation by women in races still lagged far behind men. It was thought that some women felt uncomfortable at these events. In order to provide more emotional support and to encourage women runners from the elite level on down, women-only races were established.

Kathrine Switzer knows all about this. In 1967, she ran and finished the Boston Marathon despite its ban on women participation, and after narrowly missing being thrown off the course as she ran. In 1972 she created the Avon International Women's Running Circuit, a 400-event series spanning 27 countries. She launched a second series that ran between 1998 and 2004.

Women's races are still being held, with the same goals, making it a great bucket list item for all female runners. One to check out is the Women's Run Series (https://www.womensrunseries.co.uk/).

NOTES

● RUN A WOMEN'S RACE   Date: ....

RUN IN THE GREAT ETHIOPIAN RUN

So far, all of the races listed in this chapter take place within the U.K. and U.S. That's not to detract from all of the many great races held around the world—and we'll get to some great marathons abroad in just a bit. We're going to correct that a bit right now by looking to east Africa, where a race created by the legendary Olympic champion and multiple world-record holder Haile Gebrselassie should be on your bucket list.

After returning from the 2000 Olympic Games, Gebrselassie decided that what Africa needed was not just more elite athletes, but a mass running event that could attract runners of all abilities. Thus, the Great Ethiopian Run was created—a 10K/6.2-mile race held in late November. The first edition in 2001 quickly sold out, with 10,000 registrants, and has steadily grown since. It's now the largest race in Africa, with 45,000 runners. The race has become not just a focus for elite Ethiopian runners, but also a showcase for up-and-coming runners hoping to make a name for themselves and attract the attention of sponsors. But for the thousands of other participants, it's simply a fun run and an incredible event.

If you decide to do this race, you can combine it with a trip to the high-altitude training camps to be found just outside of Addis Ababa, as we'll talk about in Chapter Seven. For information on this race, as well as other Ethiopian races, visit www.ethiopianrun.org.

NOTES

■ **RUN IN THE GREAT ETHIOPIAN RUN** Date:

RUN THE GREAT NORTH RUN

With over 60,000 participants, The Great North Run is the world's largest half marathon and a race not to be missed.

This iconic event takes place in the North East of England every year and is known for its fun and supportive atmosphere. The 13.1-mile (21.1K) course begins in Newcastle, runs over the Tyne Bridge, and finishes in the coastal town of South Shields. It was originally devised by former Olympic 10,000m bronze medalist and BBC Sport commentator Brendan Foster, who wanted to encourage and inspire runners in his home region.

Elite runners and celebrities often take part, but most people doing the race are amateurs and are raising money for charity. If you take part in The Great North Run, you can expect to be cheered on by a big crowd. Even better, the Red Arrows (the RAF aerobatics team) usually carry out a spectacular flyover during the event, making for an unforgettable, patriotic spectacle.

Spaces get snapped up early and you'll need to apply for your spot via ballot at The Great North Run website: https://www.greatrun.org/events/great-north-run/

NOTES

....
....
....
....
....
....
....
....
....
....
....
....

● **RUN THE GREAT NORTH RUN** Date: ....

CHAPTER 5

8 Epic Marathons You Need to Do

- The London Marathon *(page 95)*
- Pikes Peak Marathon *(page 97)*
- The Great Wall Marathon *(page 99)*
- Mont-Blanc Marathon *(page 101)*
- Firenze Marathon *(page 103)*
- An Indoor Marathon *(page 105)*
- Marathon des Châteaux du Médoc *(page 107)*
- The Dramathon *(page 109)*

The marathon is always a great adventure, wherever and whenever it is held. But among the many marathons held around the world, there are some that stand head and shoulders above the rest. Whether it's because of the exotic location and breathtaking scenery, or the uniquely challenging nature of the race itself, or both, these marathons should be on every runner's bucket list.

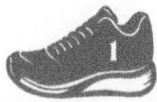

THE LONDON MARATHON

Of all the things on this bucket list, the London Marathon isn't just a must-do—it's a rite of passage.

Founded in 1981 by Olympic legends Chris Brasher and John Disley, this race has become the world's largest single-day fundraising event, raising over £1.3 billion for charity. But it's not just the numbers that make it iconic—it's the energy, the eccentricity, and the sheer magic of running through one of the greatest cities on Earth.

Held every April, the marathon covers a 26.2-mile course that begins in Blackheath and finishes triumphantly on The Mall. Along the way, runners pass some of London's most iconic landmarks, including the Tower of London and Buckingham Palace. Notably, from 1982 to 1993, the finish line was located on Westminster Bridge, but it was relocated in 1994 due to bridge repairs.

The London Marathon is famous not just for its scale, but for its vibrant atmosphere. Runners often don flamboyant costumes, and the streets are lined with some of the most enthusiastic supporters you'll ever encounter. In true London fashion, surprises abound—couples have even tied the knot mid-race, so don't be shocked if you spot a wedding dress among the crowd!

The event holds multiple world records and continues to inspire runners of all ages. According to data from Strava, the fastest participants tend to be in the 35–44 age group. And with an impressive 98 percent completion rate, it's a race that welcomes and celebrates perseverance.

NOTES

● **THE LONDON MARATHON** Date:

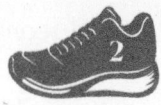

PIKES PEAK MARATHON

The good news about this race is that there's only one hill. The bad news is that it climbs steadily for almost 13 miles up to 14,005 feet.[12] From there, volunteers spin you around and point you right back downhill. If you think that it will be easier to run downhill than up, you—and your quads—will be in for a surprise.

Begun in 1956, this race starts in Manitou Springs, a Colorado town just six miles west of better-known Colorado Springs. The race director warns participants that the climb up to the half-way point might take as long as their full 26.2-mile marathon time—or more. The climb is not on the Pikes Peak Highway; instead, runners use the Barr Trail, ascending 7,815 feet on a dirt road, negotiating switchbacks as they climb.

For many participants, running turns into hiking above the tree line. Weather can also be a concern, as the mountain itself generates its own climate, meaning that what you experience at the bottom can be very different from what's going on near the summit.

If you're a flatland runner, you might be gasping for air as you shuffle to the turnaround point at the top of the mountain, but amazingly, upon turning around, your tired legs can suddenly feel fresh, and running—seemingly impossible moments earlier—might feel almost easy. But a new challenge arises at this point, as the pounding on your legs can be unmerciful as you descend and footing can be treacherous—it's common to see runners with skinned and bleeding knees, hands, and elbows.

---

12 The actual summit is slightly higher, at 14,115 feet.

When you reach the bottom and receive your finisher's medal, you may ask yourself if it seems right to even call this a marathon at all, because it feels like a different kind of event entirely. But whatever you want to call it, you will never forget it.

In addition to the marathon, there is also a separate climb-only race, known as the Pikes Peak Ascent, that is held on a different weekend. (Website: www.pikespeakmarathon.org)

NOTES

● **PIKES PEAK MARATHON** Date: ....

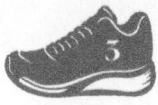

THE GREAT WALL MARATHON

It's been said that you can see the Great Wall of China from outer space. It turns out that's not true, but that doesn't detract from the Wall's grandeur. Begun in the seventh century BC, the Wall is a series of linked towers and fortifications in Northern China that were intended as a defense against various marauding nomadic tribes. Construction continued for almost two thousand years, resulting in a stone edifice that's over 21,000K (13,000 miles) long.

For runners, the Wall represents a challenge that is both irresistible and insane. Running on the Wall might look like a grand adventure, but the logistics of making this a reality can seem overwhelming. While parts of the Wall have been restored, much of it is in poor condition, and the route is far from flat; the Wall follows the undulating contours of the land that it is built on, and contains approximately 3,100 stairs.

Lucky for us, in 1999, race organizers solved the Great Wall puzzle, designing a race course northeast of Beijing that takes runners atop a section of the Wall twice, while also leading them

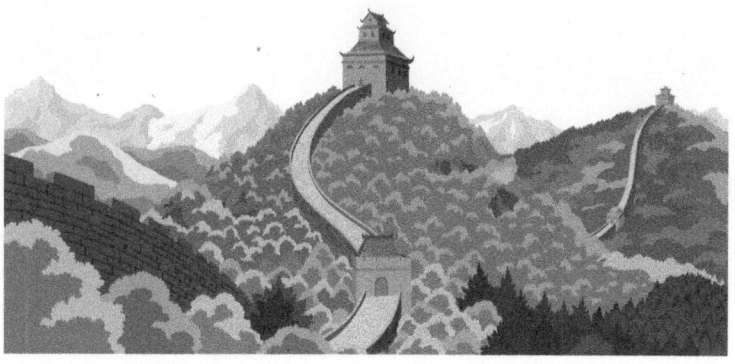

alongside and over a river, and through several villages, before crossing the finish line at the fortress of the Huangyaguan section of the Wall. While most of the race is actually run on asphalt roads, by race end, participants will have climbed 5,164 stone and brick steps on the Great Wall.

Held annually in mid-May, The Great Wall Marathon also features a half marathon, and an 8.5K/5.5 mile non-competitive fun run. There is an eight-hour time limit, starting from the release of the last of four waves of runners. Participants who miss that cutoff may continue as non-timed runners. The gate leading to the Wall will be kept open for another six hours after that, and the race officially ends two hours later—sixteen hours after the last of the waves began—at which time any participants still on the course will be transported by car to the finish line. (Website: www.great-wall-marathon.com)

NOTES

● THE GREAT WALL MARATHON   Date: ....

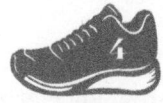

MONT-BLANC MARATHON

For trail runners, the thought of running in the French Alps is like the Holy Grail. That makes this race a dream come true.

This trail race takes place in Chamonix, located in Southeastern France, just north of Mont Blanc, the tallest peak in Western Europe and the race's namesake. The marathon is part of a collection of eight separate races held annually over a three-day period in June, attracting over 10,000 participants, making it one of the largest trail-running series in the world.

The 23K (14.3 miles) race actually came first, having been established in 1979. The marathon was added in 2003 and includes some of the same route as the shorter distance. The weekend's options also include a 3.8K/2.36 mile race, a 10K/6.2 mile race, and a 90K/55.9 mile ultra-marathon. A night-time two-person team 21K/13.1 mile race has also been added, as well as several children's events. Whichever event you choose, you are certain to be rewarded with stunning views of the Chamonix valley.

The marathon is the weekend's centerpiece and features over 8,000 total feet of elevation gain. After the in-town race starts, participants climb up to Aiguillette des Posettes and pass along a ridge for stunning views of the valley below. From there, the racecourse is an Alpine roller coaster, dropping down into the town of Vallorcine, near the border with Switzerland, and then up to the Col des Montets and the lift station at La Flégère, before dropping back down to the finish line in the center of town. There is a 10-hour time limit, and runners must make the cutoff times at each station, or they will be disqualified. Any participant who crosses past the 10-hour limit will not be timed.

You may not be able to pronounce or remember all the names of all the places you pass on the course, but you will never forget what you saw, and how hard you had to work to earn those magnificent views. (Website: www.marathonmontblanc.fr)

NOTES

● MONT-BLANC MARATHON   Date: ....

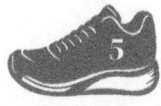

FIRENZE MARATHON

As a confirmed marathon junkie, I'm often asked which marathon is my favorite. I find that a hard question to answer because every marathon has its charms. But when push comes to shove, for me there is no city course as stunning as the Firenze (Florence) Marathon. Run in late November since 1984, this race is a wonderful tour of the city center of this ancient Italian city.

Running this race is like racing through an art history class or a museum. Participants stream through the Piazza del Duomo, past the Santa Maria del Fiore Cathedral, with its miraculous dome and its massive bronze door masterpieces. Runners also pass the historic Ponte Vecchio bridge, with stunning views of the Arno River.

The course is pancake flat, which makes it fast. But because the streets aren't closed, runners have complained about having to race through groups of pedestrians near the end of the course. That seems to me to be a small price to pay for a trip through one of the most beautiful cities in the world. And perhaps it's also for the best. If runners are forced to slow down a bit near the end, they would have some strength in their legs for after the race, so they can retrace much of the course and examine this beautiful city at a more leisurely pace. (Website: www.firenzemarathon.it/en/marathon)

NOTES

....
....
....
....
....
....
....
....
....
....
....
....
....
....

● **FIRENZE MARATHON** Date: ....

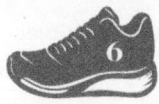

AN INDOOR MARATHON

Okay, this isn't a destination race. You will certainly not pass any points of interest on the course, and most people would probably not classify it as an epic event. Indeed, if distance running sounds repetitive and boring to you, then your head will explode when you consider this race: running between 95 and 212 laps on an indoor track.

It does sound insane, but this is a challenge that every runner should try at least once to test their mind as much as their body. Let's also not forget that there are several upsides to this event: Restrooms, gear, and refreshments are never more than a few dozen yards away, and there is no need to wonder what the weather will be on race day. And, of course, it can take place at a time of year when there are few, if any, other outdoor race options available.

Emotionally, you may find that an indoor marathon feels surprisingly similar to its outdoor cousins: Runners start off with enthusiasm, settle into their pace, manage their way through the difficult middle miles, and then hope for a second wind as they make their way to the final lap. With little on the "course" to capture your imagination, you might find that your focus turns even more inward, and your running becomes more and more automatic as the miles slip by.

The number of competitors is understandably restricted, and there are only a few of these races currently held, so if you are planning to give this a try, target it early in your schedule and keep track of application deadlines. Here are two indoor marathons for you to consider:

The Pettit Indoor Marathon takes place on a 400-meter track in Milwaukee, and is limited to 130 participants. It consists of 95.1 chip-timed laps, with a six-hour time limit. (Website: www.pettitindoormarathon.com)

The Hawk Indoor Marathon is held on a 200-meter track at Thomas Jefferson Middle School in Arlington, Virginia. Participants must cover 211 laps within a six-hour time limit. (Website: hawkindoormarathon.itsyourrace.com)

NOTES

● **AN INDOOR MARATHON** Date:

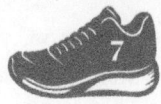

MARATHON DES CHÂTEAUX DU MÉDOC

Held every September since 1985 through the vineyards of Médoc in the Bordeaux region of Southwestern France, this race labels itself "the longest Marathon in the world." But that's not because it's longer than 26.2 miles from start to finish; it's because it's hard to run a straight line if you partake of all the wine and food that's available on the course.

Originally conceived of as a tour of wineries, it was converted into a race, but it still maintains its original focus. Along its route you will pass not just vineyards and beautiful châteaux, but 23 wine-tasting stops. And because you shouldn't partake of all that wine without some food, there is an oyster station and a steak station in the last few miles of the race.

As you might imagine, this race puts fun above performance. Runners are encouraged to wear costumes, and some 90 percent of participants choose to do so. Racers in costume will be awarded a bottle of wine upon finishing, but don't worry if you don't bring a costume; volunteers are available in the final kilometer to dab face paint on your cheeks to make sure that you, too, will be deemed to be in costume at the finish line.

The carnival atmosphere continues after the race with a party and fireworks, and, for those who want more—and who wouldn't?—there is a 10K/6.2 mile walk the next day to give racers a chance to see the region in a less hurried fashion, followed by a luncheon.

For the few days after the marathon, your legs might feel like you've finished a race, but you'll think you've just been to one of the best parties of your life. (Website: www.marathondumedoc.com/en)

NOTES

....
....
....
....
....
....
....
....
....
....
....
....
....
....
....

● **MARATHON DES CHÂTEAUX DU MÉDOC** Date: ....

THE DRAMATHON

When I first came upon this event, I thought it had something to do with the internal fights, grudges, squabbles, and knock-down, drag-out battles like my family seems to enjoy, but it turns out the root of the name isn't *"drama,"* but *"dram,"* as in a measure of whiskey.

Held in the Speyside region of Scotland, this race was conceived by a pair of friends who loved both single-malt whiskey and running, and who decided to bring their two passions together in one event. Actually, it's four events, limited to a field of 1,500 participants: The Full Dram (the marathon), the Half Dram (a half marathon), the Wee Dram (a 10K/6.2 mile run), and the We Dram (a relay).

The Full Dram begins at the Glenfarclas distillery, and covers a few hills before passing Ballindalloch Castle and continuing on the mostly level foot trail along the river Spey, joining up with the other races along the way. Fall foliage is in full display as the course travels along an old railway line, with just three miles on paved roads. It passes several more distilleries, including the beautiful modern Dalmunach Distillery, on its way to a gradual uphill slope to the finish line at the Glenfiddich Distillery in Dufftown.

Depending on which distance you ran, you'll be greeted with a corresponding number of miniatures from the distilleries that you passed, a Glencairn Crystal tasting glass with the race logo, and a unique finisher's medal made from a whiskey barrel stave. The drinking is optional, but the breathtaking course and memories are for everyone. (Website: www.thedramathon.com)

NOTES

....
....
....
....
....
....
....
....
....
....
....
....
....
....
....
....
....
....
....

● **THE DRAMATHON** Date: ....

CHAPTER 6

7 Runs in the Footsteps of Giants

- Run the Athens Marathon *(page 112)*
- Run on an Ancient Racetrack *(page 114)*
- Run on Hayward Field, University of Oregon *(page 117)*
- Run in Stockholm Olympic Stadium, Sweden *(page 119)*
- Run on the Sir Roger Bannister Athletics Track *(page 121)*
- Run in Iten, Kenya *(page 123)*
- Run in Addis Ababa, Ethiopia *(page 125)*

The sport of running has a history. Ancient legends tell stories of incredible running feats and races, and modern heroes perform equally legendary feats. While other sports may have illustrious histories as well, few offer the opportunity to participate in a sport exactly where the legendary heroes performed. Only running can really provide that experience. You may not be able to square up in the batter's box at Wrigley Field or take a jump shot on the basketball court at Madison Square Garden, but you can still run in the footsteps of your running heroes, because many of these historic courses are available for you to experience yourself. So, lace up your shoes, and let's dream a little dream of running.

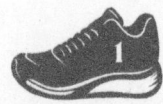

RUN THE ATHENS MARATHON

This marathon race was created in 1896 for the first modern Olympic Games, but the legend of the marathon goes back over two thousand years.

According to the ancient historians Herodotus and Plutarch, Greek runners were used as messengers during the Greco-Persian wars, which took place from 499 to 449 BC. According to legend, after a small Athenian army defeated a much larger Persian force on the plains of Marathon in 490 BC, the messenger Pheidippides raced from the site of the battle to Athens, some 25 miles away, to deliver news of the victory. He declared, "Nike!" meaning, "We are victorious!" and then collapsed and died.

Is the story true? Perhaps. The battle certainly took place. True or not, Pheidippides' legendary run was the inspiration for the modern race, which takes its name from the battle site. Every marathon race can trace its origin back to that run, but none more so than the Athens Marathon, which aims to follow Pheidippides' route.

Race participants begin at Marathon and circle a giant burial mound, in which the bodies of those ancient warriors were laid to rest. Runners make their way on paved city roads, but in their imaginations, they may be running on dusty dirt in sandals.

This is the course that was used in the very first modern Olympic Games in 1896, for which the modern marathon was invented, and again when the Olympics returned to Athens in 2004. Race participants can finish their run just as those Olympians did, with a lap within the ancient marble stadium, which we will talk about next. (Website: www.athensauthenticmarathon.gr)

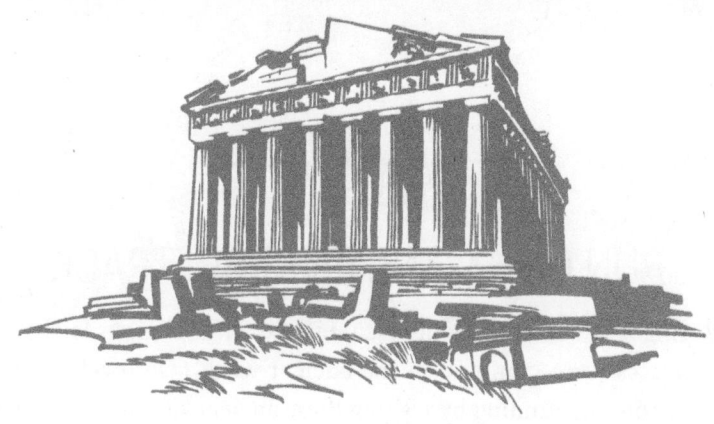

NOTES

● RUN THE ATHENS MARATHON   Date:..........................

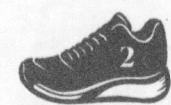

RUN ON AN ANCIENT RACETRACK

Racing is as old as mankind itself. Linked with religious festivals, footraces were common in the ancient world. Get back to the deep roots of running by visiting these ancient sites and running in the footsteps of our ancestors.

PANATHENAIC STADIUM, ATHENS, GREECE. The only stadium in the world built entirely of marble, it dates back to around 330 BC, when it was host to the Panathenaic Games. It was abandoned around the fourth century with the rise of Christianity, but it was later excavated and put back into service for the opening and closing ceremonies of the first modern Olympic Games in 1896, and again when the Olympic Games returned to Athens in 2004.

Located in central modern Athens, the Panathenaic Stadium has been the finishing point for the annual Athens Marathon. This is, literally, where long-distance road racing began, and you don't have to run a marathon to experience it yourself.

CIRCUS MAXIMUS. Built in central Rome in the sixth century BC as a venue for chariot races, this was the first and largest stadium of ancient Rome. It measured 2,037 feet in length and 387 feet in width and could accommodate over 150,000 spectators. It was the site for *ludi*, the public games connected to Roman religious festivals. Varying in duration and complexity, the ludi eventually were held on 135 days of the year, and in addition to chariot races and gladiator matches, they featured long-distance footraces.

Over time, other venues, such as the Coliseum, started to draw events away from the Circus Maximus, and with the rise of Christianity, the ludi themselves fell out of favor. The last known races were held at the Circus Maximus in AD 549. In the years that followed, the venue fell into decay, as the flood-prone area was gradually covered in soil and debris. Over the following centuries, the area was used for housing, as a market, and in the nineteenth century, as the site of gas works. Stone from the ancient structures was removed and repurposed for other buildings. Excavations in the twentieth century uncovered some of the original stadium, including lower sections of seating and an outer portico. It now serves as a free public park, with tours available to help visitors interpret the site. Visit the site for yourself and run along its paths. With a little imagination, you can envision what it might have been like to race there, in front of some of the largest sporting event crowds in history.

NOTES

....
....
....
....
....
....
....
....
....
....
....
....
....
....

● **RUN ON AN ANCIENT RACETRACK** Date: ....

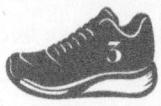

RUN ON HAYWARD FIELD, UNIVERSITY OF OREGON

Most runners tend to focus their interest in running on their own training and racing, giving little thought to the sport as such. I would bet with confidence that few participants in a big race know or care who the winners are. Occasionally a few elite runners burst out onto the big stage, but most elite runners toil in relative obscurity.

Perhaps that's how it should be. We run for our own health and well-being, alone or with a few friends. Elite runners are almost always strangers, their achievements don't have anything to do with our own love of running and what running brings to our lives.

But still, there are some places that are drenched in running history, and simply being there can instill motivation and a sense of being part of something bigger than ourselves.

Hayward Field is one of these places. Located on the campus of the University of Oregon in the town of Eugene, it was built in 1919 for football and has been the home of track and field teams since 1921, when a cinder track was added.

Named for longtime coach William "Colonel Bill" Hayward, this site is also known as TrackTown USA, since so much of the history of American track and field played out on its 400-meter oval track. It has been a frequent host to national championships and Olympic trials, and the list of runners who competed there for the fabled Oregon teams is a who's who of running: Steve Prefontaine, Alberto Salazar, Galen Rupp, Kenny Moore, and Nike founder Phil Knight.

The track and the grandstands have been replaced and modernized, but the spirit of running lives on this hallowed ground. Do a few laps there and soak it up.

While you're there, look for the statue of Bill Bowerman, the famed longtime coach of the University's track team, and a cofounder of the Nike sports brand. His likeness holds a stopwatch as he stands astride a waffle iron, commemorating his experiments in making custom shoes. He reportedly poured hot rubber onto his wife's waffle iron to create the outsole he wanted for his shoes, and in doing so, passed into legend.

NOTES

● **RUN ON HAYWARD FIELD, UNIVERSITY OF OREGON** Date:

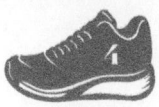

RUN IN STOCKHOLM OLYMPIC STADIUM, SWEDEN

The 1912 Olympics, in Stockholm, Sweden, became a showcase for one of the greatest all-around athletes the world has ever seen, Jim Thorpe.

A member of the Sac and Fox First Peoples tribes, Thorpe was already a star baseball player and an All-American collegiate football player as a running back, defensive back, placekicker and punter when he decided to train in track and field for the upcoming Games. In Stockholm, he set records on the way to winning gold in both the pentathlon and the decathlon. When presenting Thorpe with his awards, King Gustav V declared, "You, sir, are the greatest athlete in the world."[13] Thorpe returned to the United States as a hero and was the star attraction in a ticker tape parade down Broadway in New York City.

Visiting the old Olympic stadium now is like walking back in time. You walk through the brick archway and marvel at the wooden spectator stands. Looking onto the field, you see a track with modern surfacing. You may see other runners going through their workouts, but ignore them as you do a few laps, while trying to imagine what it was like over a century ago to be in that stadium, or even on that track, when Jim Thorpe amazed the world.

---

13 Thorpe was stripped of his medals shortly after the Olympics for violating unfair rules regarding amateurism by accepting money for playing baseball. That decision was finally reversed over a century later, in 2022, when he was declared the sole winner of those events.

NOTES

....
....
....
....
....
....
....
....
....
....
....
....
....
....
....
....

- **RUN IN STOCKHOLM OLYMPIC STADIUM, SWEDEN** Date:..

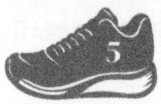

RUN ON THE SIR ROGER BANNISTER ATHLETICS TRACK

Also known as the Oxford University track, or the Iffley Road track. On this hallowed ground in Oxford, England, one of the seminal sporting moments of the twentieth century took place on May 6, 1954, when Roger Bannister became the first person in history to run a mile in under four minutes.

Before Bannister accomplished his great feat, it was widely considered impossible. Many people believed that anyone attempting it would risk having their heart or lungs explode. But on that day, 25-year-old Bannister, a medical student at the time, recruited two other runners to pace him through the first three-quarters of the mile in under three minutes, and then blazed through the final lap alone to cross the tape in 3:59:4. He collapsed after finishing, but quickly recovered, and walked right into the history books.

Since that fateful day over 70 years ago, 1,755 athletes have matched Bannister's feat. The current record is 3:43:13, set by Moroccan athlete Hicham El Guerrouj in 1999. But, of course, there's nothing like the first time. When Bannister accomplished the impossible, he destroyed the mental barrier that had stopped so many other runners from achieving that goal.

The track itself dates back to 1876, when the University of Oxford decided to build a new track to replace another one that it had built nearby nine years earlier, but which had frequently been flooded. In 1948, Bannister was a 19-year-old student when he was elected president of the Oxford University Athletic Club. He arranged to have the old track replaced with a new, modern track, which was unveiled in 1950. This was the track on which he made history.

Since then, the track has been refurbished three times, most recently in 2007, when it was renamed the Sir Roger Bannister Athletics Track. Bannister passed away in 2018, but the track named for him is open to the public. Step onto it and make history of your own.

NOTES

● **RUN ON THE SIR ROGER BANNISTER ATHLETICS TRACK** Date: ....

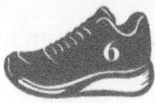

RUN IN ITEN, KENYA

Kenyan runners are legendary among endurance athletes. While the names—often unusual to American ears and hard for us to pronounce—may change, the place of Kenyans at the top of every major marathon finisher's list seems to be a constant.

This history of Kenyan racing exceptionalism may have its roots in many causes—the epigenetic effect of living at high altitude, the poverty that creates a burning desire to achieve, the Kenyan culture of running—but whatever its origin, Kenyan racing dominance all starts here, in a small town in the Kenyan highlands, and the edge of the Rift Valley.

Situated at an elevation of 7,900 feet above sea level, this town name comes from a corruption of "Hill Ten," the designation of a local rock formation that was named in 1883. But this town of just over 42,000 people is more accurately known as "The Home of Champions," and for good reason. The list of athletes who came from here or trained here is a who's who of elite runners. New York City and three-time Boston Marathon champion Ibrahim Hussein, Olympic gold medalist Peter Rono and silver medalist Wilson Kipketer, and world champions Edna Kiplagat, Mary Jepkosgei Keitany, Lornah Kiplagat, and a host of others.

World Athletics has awarded Iten a plaque recognizing it as a World Athletics Heritage Landmark, and elite runners come here for the High Altitude Training Center, founded in 1999. Come for a visit and join in for workouts with the locals. Don't be ashamed if you can't keep up; just enjoy the beautiful natural surroundings, the running culture, the food, and the friendly people. Whether you make your own arrangements, or travel with a running tour group, this can be a running trip of a lifetime. (Website: www.traininkenya.com)

NOTES

....
....
....
....
....
....
....
....
....
....
....
....
....
....
....
....
....

● **RUN IN ITEN, KENYA** Date: ....

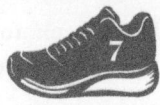

RUN IN ADDIS ABABA, ETHIOPIA

If there are any runners who can challenge the elite Kenyans, it's the Ethiopians. Sharing a friendly but fierce rivalry going back decades, the Kenyan and Ethiopian runners trade first-place finishes and world records back and forth among themselves like party favors.

Much of the success enjoyed by the Ethiopian elite runners is based on circumstances that they share with the Kenyan runners: living and training at high altitude, having a culture of running, and viewing running as a way to escape poverty.

Addis Ababa is the capital city of Ethiopia, and it offers runners a wide range of unforgettable training options in the city and nearby. Within the city, you can train on the legendary Legetafo Track, a winding 400-meter dirt loop that is open to the public and attracts hundreds of runners daily. There is also Meskel Square, where an outdoor amphitheater provides the setting for a stair workout for local runners.

Just outside the city, you can do hill runs along a eucalyptus forest in the village of Sululta. You should also plan a visit to the high altitude Yaya Athletics Village in the Entoto Mountains, which was founded by champion marathoner Haile Gebrselassie and features running and training facilities.

The village of Bekoji also belongs on your must-see list. Known as the "Town of Runners," it is the home village of champion runners Derartu Tulu, Fatuma Roba, and Kenenisa Bekele.

You may time your visit to Ethiopia to coincide with the Great Ethiopian Run, a 10K race founded by legendary Ethiopian running champion Haile Gebrselassie. For more information on this event, see Chapter Four.

Your visit to Ethiopia will be breathtaking—literally!—and it will fill you with enough inspiring memories to power many miles of running once you're back home.

NOTES

⬤ **RUN IN ADDIS ABABA, ETHIOPIA** Date:..............................

CHAPTER 7

7 Ultra-Marathons, Stage Races, and Relays You Need to Try

- Marathon des Sables *(page 128)*
- Himalayan 100-Mile Stage Race and Mt. Everest Challenge Marathon *(page 131)*
- The Barkley Marathons *(page 134)*
- JFK 50 Mile *(page 137)*
- Western States Endurance Run *(page 138)*
- Comrades Marathon *(page 141)*
- Providence Hood and Portland to Coast Relay *(page 144)*

It's a famous axiom among a select group of runners: "Any idiot can run a marathon, but it takes a special kind of idiot to run an ultra." When a mountain has been conquered, it is perhaps just human nature to look for another taller peak to tackle. Once the marathon beast has been subdued, some runners wonder if they could go even farther. For them, there is the ultra-marathon.

Defined as any distance that exceeds the standard marathon distance of 26.2 miles, the ultra-marathon is typically raced at 50K, 50 miles, 100K, and 100 miles. Others are raced in time rather than distance, as in the 24-hour races, where runners are challenged to cover as much ground as they could in the allotted time.

Some ultras cannot fit into these neat limits and sprawl out over odd distances. Other long distances can't even be contained in one day of running and are broken up into timed stages over several days. Still more require teams of runners to work together to conquer courses that are hundreds of miles long.

All of these races challenge the body, mind, and spirit. They are the unforgettable, often once-in-a-lifetime challenges that, for many runners, are the final word in bucket list achievements.

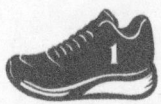

MARATHON DES SABLES

You wonder sometimes who is crazier: the people who conceived of and organized this event, or the participants. It's a chicken and egg debate, and I suppose it hardly matters. The end result is the same: mass insanity.

The *Marathon des Sables* (MdS) translates into "Marathon of the Sands." It is a seven-day, 160-mile run across the Sahara Desert in southern Morocco. It was dreamed up in 1984 by Patrick Bauer, who had just hiked 214 miles across the desert alone. He wondered whether he could create an event based on his experience. Two years later, the MdS was born.

In accordance with Bauer's solo experience, the goal of the MdS is self-sufficiency. Participants must carry all of the supplies they will use for the race—all the food they will consume, and clothing and gear they will use, for the entire event. The race provides tent accommodations, and water at each morning's start, but after that, the runners are on their own, except for emergency support.

It's hard to fully prepare for the conditions that runners will encounter in this event. Wind, blowing sand, fearsome blisters, and searing heat are just some of the challenges that participants will face. After registering for the race, participants will receive regular emails containing tips that are specific for this event, such as conditioning the feet to be more blister resistant, choosing the right ankle gaiters to keep sand out of your shoes, and picking the right pack to run with.

Needless to say, this race is not about speed. But still, participants need to keep an eye on pace. If they fall too far behind, they will encounter the dreaded camel. Acting as a sweep vehicle, a race official atop a camel trails the pack of racers. If the camel passes you, you are disqualified, and your race is over.

The MdS has expanded to include a shorter-stage race, as well as events in other locations, but for many, there's nothing like the legendary original race. Finish this race, and you will believe that you can truly do anything that you set your mind to. (Website: www.marathondessables.com)

NOTES

● **MARATHON DES SABLES** Date:..................................

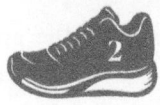

HIMALAYAN 100-MILE STAGE RACE AND MT. EVEREST CHALLENGE MARATHON

There are some races that provide magical moments, when you look around and realize how lucky you are to be where you are, doing what you're doing.

This is one of those races. It was created in 1991 by the charismatic C. S. Pandey, who then, as now, led climbing groups up into his beloved mountains. In 1991 he was challenged by a female athlete to create a route that she could run, with his support. Pandey rose to the challenge and has been the race director of this event ever since.

This is a five-day event that will leave you literally gasping, both in awe and for air. An international group of 20 to 60 runners gather in the airport in Delhi for a brief overnight stay before continuing on by air north to Darjeeling. After some sightseeing among the tea plantations, a mountaineering museum, and a zoo

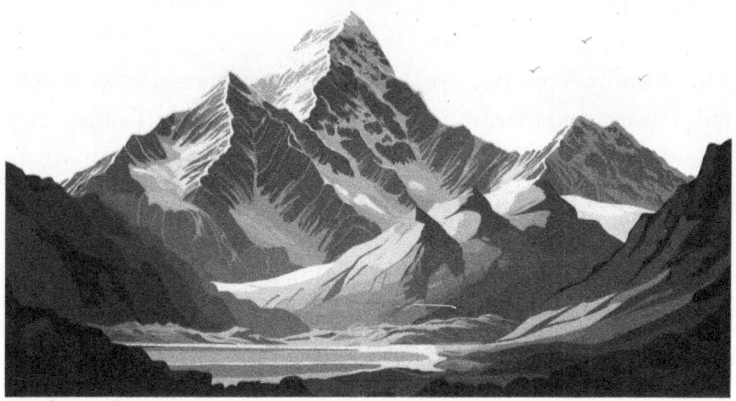

with exotic Himalayan animals, the group heads up by bus to begin the real work—the start of the race in the small town of Maneybhanjang, at 6,600 feet above sea level.

At the race start, runners are greeted by local children, who drape them in scarves for good luck and cheer them on as the race begins. The runners stream through town but then mostly walk as they ascend 6,000 feet over the course of 24 miles, to the Sandakphu encampment.

Sunrise, the next morning at 12,000 feet above sea level, greets participants with an amazing panoramic view of Mt. Everest, Lhotse, Makalu, and Kanchenjunga—four of the five highest mountains in the world (only K2 is missing), before they head out for a 20-mile out-and-back run. On day three, runners head out the same way as previously, but continue on instead of turning back, descending to the town of Rimbik. This day's run is 26 miles (likely a bit more), and serves as the Mt. Everest Marathon Challenge, a race-within-a-race. The final two days of racing return runners to paved roads, as they continue to descend, making their way through lush tropical foliage and past small villages, finishing where they began. Afterwards, Mr. Pandey and crew host a celebration dinner and awards ceremony for the participants, who by now have changed from a bunch of individual runners into a community.

This is a fully supported event, with trailing vans and well-stocked aid stations, and there are no age or time limits. Mr. Pandey truly believes that anyone can complete this event, and he strives to provide enough support to make this true. Participants can opt to tackle the full 100-mile trek, a 100K race, or just the marathon. All meals, lodging, and connections are included, along with sightseeing in Darjeeling.

If an event can be personified by one individual, it is this race, and the person is Mr. Pandey. His enthusiasm for the event, the land, the people, and his racers and visitors is palpable and infectious. He is your crazy uncle, your doting grandfather, your best friend, and your personal cheerleader all wrapped up in one. Without Mr. Pandey, there is no race, and with him, it's an occasion not to be missed.

I enjoyed this event so much that after completing it, I returned a decade later for a second run, and I wouldn't rule out a third trip someday. On both trips, I opted to add a one-day side trip offered by Mr. Pandey from Delhi to Agra to see the fabled Taj Mahal. (Website: www.himalayan.com)

NOTES

● **HIMALAYAN STAGE RACE AND MT. EVEREST CHALLENGE MARATHON** Date:

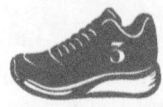

THE BARKLEY MARATHONS

This event is widely viewed as the most challenging foot race in the world. "Craziest" might be another apt description, and for good reason. There is nothing easy about it, from registering for it, to starting it, and, if you are lucky enough, to finishing it.

First, a bit of history. James Earl Ray, who had assassinated Martin Luther King, Jr., was being held in Brushy Mountain State Penitentiary in Morgan County, Tennessee, when he managed to escape in 1977. After a massive manhunt, he was recaptured two days later after only making it eight miles through the thick woods.

Gary Cantrell (aka Lazarus Lake) thought he could have done much better. In fact, he believed he would have been able to cover 100 miles in that time in the hills around the prison. And thus, in 1986, the Barkley Marathons were born.[14] It's a 100-mile five-loop ultra-marathon, with a "fun run" ultra-marathon option of 60 miles/three loops.

Okay, let's talk registration. There's a race cap of 40 men and women, but there are no prerequisites. In fact, race bib #1 is reserved for the person viewed as least likely to succeed, known as "the Human Sacrifice." The fee is $1.60. You read that right. A little over a buck and a half. Plus, you'll need to submit an essay describing your qualifications, or lack thereof, in as interesting and witty a fashion as possible. All of this is to be sent to the race

---

14 The origin of the name is a mystery, which fits right in with the nature of this race.

director, but there is no official website, and details on how to actually register are hard to find. Good luck there.

If you do manage to register, you may receive a letter of condolences from Cantrell, which means you've been accepted. As a participant, you are expected to pay another fee: a donation of some article of clothing, and first-timers are also asked to bring a license plate from their home state.

The race itself takes place on the weekend nearest April Fool's Day, within Frozen Head State Park, in Wartburg, Tennessee, close to the prison. Unsurprisingly, there is no trail map. Runners must complete five loops to be declared a finisher, but the course is hard to follow, and there is a total elevation gain of 60,000 feet—more than twice the height of Mt. Everest.

The race begins one hour after Cantrell blows a conch shell, which can happen at any time between midnight and noon on race day. Participants then have 60 hours to complete the race, which is composed of two laps of the course in one direction, two laps in the other direction, and either way on the last loop. Runners certify that they have completed each loop by tearing a page out of a book at the official checkpoint. If you are missing a page, you don't get credit for the loop.

Concerned? You should be. Very few participants manage to complete the race. As of 2024, only 17 runners managed this feat. All the others were greeted by the playing of "Taps" when they dropped out. But completing even one loop is considered a feat to be proud of.

For more information, you can consult numerous articles online, or the book *Tales From Out There: The Barkley Marathons, the World's Toughest Trail Race*,[15] and two aptly-named documentaries:

---

15 By Frozen Ed Furtaw (CreateSpace, 2010).

The Barkley Marathons: The Race That Eats Its Young (2014) and *Where Dreams Go To Die* (2017).

If all of this intrigues you, then you are a deeply disturbed person, and I view you as a kindred spirit. I haven't tackled the Barkley myself, but it's on my list.

NOTES

....
....
....
....
....
....
....
....
....
....
....
....
....
....

● **THE BARKLEY MARATHONS** Date: ....

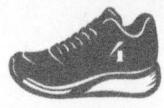

JFK 50 MILE

This ultra-marathon was established in the spring of 1963 in response to President John F. Kennedy's call for Americans to improve their fitness. Kennedy had specifically challenged his military officers to meet the requirement that President Teddy Roosevelt had set down over a half century earlier: to cover 50 miles on foot within 20 hours to keep their commission.

Thus, the JFK Challenge was born. Although it was envisioned as a military event, it immediately attracted not just commissioned officers, but NCOs and civilians as well.

After President Kennedy was assassinated that November, many events that had sprung up in the wake of Kennedy's call to the nation were canceled. But not the 50 Mile Challenge. It changed its name to the JFK Memorial 50, and it is now the oldest, and largest, ultra-marathon in the United States.

The race starts in the town of Boonsboro, Maryland, and after a few miles on the road, it heads onto the Appalachian Trail for 13 rocky, hilly miles, then drops down onto the much flatter Chesapeake & Ohio Canal Towpath trail for a full marathon run. (See Chapter Twelve for more on both trails.) From there, it's 8.4 miles on paved roads to the finish line in Williamsport, Maryland.

Finishing any ultra-marathon is a huge accomplishment, but with its history, the JFK 50 is a special one. Since it's held in late November, you will be starting in the dark, and in all likelihood, you will also be finishing in the dark. When your friends ask you what you did that Sunday, you could honestly tell them that you ran *all day*. (Website: www.jfk50mile.org)

NOTES

● JFK 50 MILE Date:..

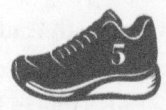

WESTERN STATES ENDURANCE RUN

The oldest and arguably the most prestigious of all American ultra-marathons, this 100.2-mile race takes place on the last weekend of June on the trails of California's Sierra Nevada mountains.

Its origins date back to a 24-hour horse-riding event called the Tevis Cup. In 1972, twenty soldiers attempted to cover the course on foot, starting one day before the horses. In 1974, legendary ultra-marathoner Gordy Ainsleigh became the first person to complete the course in under 24 hours. In 1977, the race became official, dubbed the Western States Endurance Run. In 1978, the Western States separated from the Tevis Cup, moved to June, and added aid stations.

Over the years, the course has changed slightly. Today, it covers the same route that was established in 1986. It starts at the Palisades Tahoe ski resort, crosses the Foresthill Divide and the American River Canyon, where runners will have to wade across the river using a guide rope, and finishes in Auburn, California. Participants can expect to encounter very rugged terrain, ascending a total of more than 18,000 feet and descending almost 23,000 feet before crossing the finish line. Temperatures can vary between 20 degrees Fahrenheit up to over 100, and there is often snow in the passes.

Today, the Western States Endurance Run is one of the four races that make up the "Grand Slam of Ultra-Running."[16] The list of finishers is a who's who of the greatest ultra runners, including Ann Trason (fourteen victories), Scott Jurek (seven consecutive victories), and Tim Twietmeyer (25 race finishes, including five victories).

Beyond the difficulty of the race itself, simply getting a race number is a challenge. Applicants must have run one of the qualifying ultra-marathons within the designated time period, as listed

---

16 The others in the club are the Vermont 100 Endurance Run, the Wasatch Front 100 Mile Endurance Run, and the Leadville Trail 100 Run. Any one of these races could also be on your bucket list, and completing the Grand Slam could be the ultimate goal.

on the Western States website. Because the race is held on environmentally sensitive trails within a park, the total number of participants is limited.

For these reasons, running the Western States often takes years to plan and prepare for, but for ultra-marathoners, this is the Holy Grail, and there is no substitute. (Website: www.wser.org)

NOTES

....
....
....
....
....
....
....
....
....
....
....
....
....
....
....
....

● **WESTERN STATES ENDURANCE RUN** Date: ....

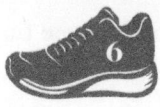

COMRADES MARATHON

Don't be fooled by the name "marathon" attached to this race. In the world of ultra-marathoning, this is the Big One. Established in 1921 by a South African World War I veteran to honor his fallen comrades, this event is the world's largest and oldest ultra. It is held in the KwaZulu-Natal province of South Africa, and its history spans the Second World War and the fall of apartheid.

Comrades is a point-to-point course, running 88K/55 miles from Pietermaritzburg to the seaside town of Durban. Unlike other races, the Comrades' course flips every year, from the "up" course finishing in Pietermaritzburg, to the "down" course in Durban. But whichever direction you run, you will have plenty of hills to contend with.

The race field is capped at 25,000, and slots are snapped up very quickly. To enter, you must submit proof that you've run a qualifying race—a marathon or longer—faster than the designated minimum times. The course passes beautiful acacia trees and flows from town to town, climbing many named hills, and has a stadium finish. But it's the field of runners that really makes the race.

It's hard to describe exactly how exciting the atmosphere is at Comrades. When I ran it, I was with a pack of runners nearing the end of the race when they spontaneously began singing "Shosholoza," the tribal work song that was traditionally sung by gold miners. The song's name roughly translates into "going forward," or "make way for the next man," and it has come to represent support for any struggle. Over the years, it became the unofficial national anthem of South Africa. Hearing this song as I labored with my fellow runners toward the finish line is still one of the most unforgettable moments of my life.

The Comrades Marathon is not just a great experience; it is also very much a competitive event. Most races offer categories for first-, second-, and third-place finishers, and finisher medals for the rest of the runners who complete the course. Not so at Comrades, where you can strive to qualify for one of nine different medals. From the bottom up, they are:

- The Vic Clapham Finisher's Medal—for a sub-12-hour finish time, this copper medal is named after the race founder.
- The Bronze Medal—for a sub-11-hour finish time.
- The Robert Mtshali Medal—for a sub-10-hour finish time, this medal is made of titanium, and is named for the first black runner, who unofficially finished the race in 1935. This medal was introduced in 2019.
- The Bill Rowan Medal—for a sub-9-hour finish time. This medal has an outer silver ring and a bronze center, and is named for the race's first winner, who won in 1921 in a time of 8:59.
- The Silver Medal—for a sub-7.5-hour finish time. This is the medal that has been around the longest, having been given to all finishers at the first race in 1921. It was the only medal until the gold medal was introduced in 1931.
- The Isavel Roche-Kelly Medal—named for the first woman to break the 7.5-hour mark, this medal is awarded to women only who finish outside the top ten but under 7 hours. It has a gold outer ring and a silver center.
- The Wally Hayward Medal—awarded to runners who finish in less than 6 hours but outside the top ten, it also has a gold outer ring and silver center. It's named for the five-time

winner of the race, who was also, later, the oldest finisher of the race, completing it at age 80 in 10 hours 58 minutes.
- The Gold Medal—awarded to the first 10 men and women to finish the race.
- The Back-to-Back Medal—awarded to runners who complete the race in consecutive years.

This range of awards gives runners many goals to shoot for, with added prestige for each rung of the medal ladder they can climb. But be aware that the finish can be brutal: The time limits are strictly enforced, and runners who don't complete the race within 12 hours are considered non-finishers, even if they are just a few feet from the finish line when the bell tolls for them. Spectators cheer on runners as the seconds count down, and groan with those who just miss completing the race. But the fear of missing the cutoff just makes crossing the line all the sweeter. (Website: www.comrades.com)

NOTES

. . . .

. . . .

. . . .

. . . .

● COMRADES MARATHON Date: . . . .

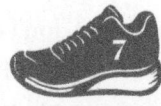

PROVIDENCE HOOD AND PORTLAND TO COAST RELAY

A relay is a completely different kind of racing experience than any other. When you compete in a relay, you are part of a team, working with other runners to achieve a joint goal. But long-distance relays aren't the pretty affairs that you might recall seeing at track meets or the Olympic Games, where runners sprint around neat tracks, passing a baton off from runner to runner, until the entire distance is covered in a few minutes.

There are some moderate-distance relays, such as those included in a marathon, where each member runs one or more legs of the race to complete the entire 26.2-mile distance. Long-distance relays are far more epic, requiring each member in teams of as many as 12 runners to race three times during the course of the event, with one of these legs taking place in the dark of night, usually covering a total distance of about 200 miles.

These events are physically and logistically challenging. Teams break down into two squads, traveling in two separate, fully stocked vans. That means that all racers have to pay for travel to the event, race entry, rental of two vans, and all the food and supplies they will need for the event.

Once the race begins, each squad of six runners in each team will rotate through their assigned legs, after which the other van will take over to complete the next six legs. This will give the first crew a long break to rest and recover before the next rotation takes place. This switch occurs three times, with each runner doing a total of about 16 miles before the team triumphantly crosses the finish line.

This is one of those instances in which the parts add up to more than the whole. While most long-distance runners don't have any significant problem with completing a 16-mile run, a relay is actually three separate races for each runner, which is a completely different animal. Each runner has to calculate what their pace should be for each leg, taking into account that they will have a break of six hours or so between each of their races. During that time, runners will try to eat and rest, catching whatever sleep they can, as they prepare for their next assigned leg.

If this seems complicated, the reality is even harder than it sounds. Getting the nutrition right can be the most vexing issue. You will want to fully refuel after each leg so that you are fully energized for your next race-within-the-race, but if you eat and drink too much, you can experience sluggishness and stomach upset when running.

Resting is also difficult, as there is not enough time to get restorative sleep between your racing assignments. Basically, everyone will be taking catnaps during the course of the nearly 24-hour event and will feel like zombies by the end.

The course itself presents additional challenges. In addition to any hills that racers have to climb, the course is not closed to traffic, which makes it unlike most other races that you have run. There will be signs along the way directing runners, and volunteers on site to help steer the runners in the right direction, but as the race field stretches out, you may find you are out on your own for miles at a time.

It was during moments like these that I realized my capacity for remembering race directions was limited to about three turns at a time. After that, I would have to consult my race map. This became especially challenging when running in the dark, especially in rural areas. If I was lucky, my team van would be nearby and could give me guidance, or I could work with other runners nearby to make sure we were all on course.

The handoff from runner to runner can also create challenges. Here, there isn't the fear of a dropped baton, as happens with track relays. Instead, there is the concern that the next runner won't be at the connection point in time for the switch. For runners who have pushed themselves to run their leg as hard as they can in order to help the team achieve its goal, it can be very frustrating to arrive at their endpoint only to find the next runner isn't ready to run.

The solution to this problem is that the team has to work together to make sure each runner knows approximately where the active runner is on the course, and be ready to run at the handoff area when the prior runner is nearing their finish. Runners in the active van will need to keep an eye on their runners and talk with the runners in the resting van to update them on the team's position. This might seem simple enough to accomplish, but add in sleep deprivation, physical fatigue, and the darkness of night, and things get trickier.

With all the challenges and expense involved in doing this event, you may wonder if it's really worth doing. The answer is a resounding YES. When all of these challenges are overcome, and the entire team joins at the finish line to celebrate their achievement, you will feel a sense of satisfaction different from—and perhaps greater than—any race finish you achieved on your own. Together, you and your team have achieved something special, and have created a bond that is rare in our sport.

The most famous of these races is the Providence Hood and Portland to Coast Relay, known as the Mother of All Relays. It is the largest relay race in the world, with 12,600 participants. Founded in 1982, the race usually sells out on the same day that registration opens.

The race takes place at the end of August, starting at the Timberline Lodge on the slopes of Mount Hood, the tallest mountain in Oregon, and travels 198 miles through Portland and the Oregon Coast Range to the finish line in the beachside town of Seaside. Along the way, runners will encounter paved roads, sidewalks, multi-use trails, and gravel roads. There are flat sections, and also ascents and descents. The race begins at 3 a.m., with runners sent off in staggered waves. There is a 36-hour time limit.

There are other distance options available on race weekend, but for the complete experience, there is nothing like participating in the full Providence Hood and Portland to Coast. (Website: www.hoodtocoast.com)

NOTES

....

....

....

....
....
....
....
....
....
....
....
....
....
....
....
....
....

- **PROVIDENCE HOOD AND PORTLAND TO COAST RELAY** Date: ....

CHAPTER 8

10 Oddball Race Ideas

- [ ] Participate in a Color Run *(page 150)*
- [ ] Do a Bubble Run *(page 151)*
- [ ] Run a Zombie Race *(page 153)*
- [ ] Run a Beer Race *(page 154)*
- [ ] Run a Mud Run/Obstacle Course Race *(page 155)*
- [ ] Tackle the Empire State Building Run-Up *(page 157)*
- [ ] Run in Fancy Dress *(page 159)*
- [ ] Aim to Finish Last in a Race *(page 160)*
- [ ] Start a Race in Last Place *(page 162)*
- [ ] Do the Rocky Run Challenge *(page 163)*

Running is serious business for many of us, but that doesn't mean we can't sometimes loosen up a bit and have some fun. All runners find at some point that running has become too much of a chore, and that racing feels like an obligation. When that happens, we need to take a break from all that and get back to just having fun. One sure way to put a smile back on your face and a bounce in your step is to try these bucket list runs.

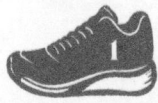

PARTICIPATE IN A COLOR RUN

Billing itself as "the Happiest 5K on the Planet," this race aims to add some color to your life. Literally. It is not a competition; the event is untimed, and no winners are declared. Instead, runners wear white clothing, which serves as a canvas when they are doused head to toe with colored powder at each of five stations along the course.

By the end of the 5K, every runner looks like a rainbow, but the fun doesn't end at the finish line. From there, participants continue on to the Finish Festival, which is a party with music, dancing, photo ops, activity booths, and yes, more color bombs. Created in 2011, the Color Run bills itself as a catalyst for a fitter lifestyle, as more than half of all of its participants are first-time 5K runners. They must be doing something right, because the race has grown to be the largest race series in the world, with events in over 50 countries, drawing over eight million total participants. (Website: www.thecolorrun.com)

NOTES

....
....
....
....
....
....
....
....
....
....
....
....
....
....
....
....

● **PARTICIPATE IN A COLOR RUN** Date:..............................

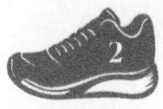

DO A BUBBLE RUN

This race is exactly what it sounds like: Participants run through a fog of colored bubbles. Imagine a car wash meeting a bubble bath, and you get the idea. But this run is strictly for fun: It's untimed. Participants are encouraged to take their time and play.

Bubble Run events are held all across the country. To find one near you—or someplace that you'd like to travel to, visit https://bubble-rush.com/events/

NOTES

● **DO A BUBBLE RUN** Date:..................................

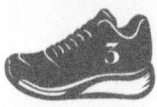

RUN A ZOMBIE RACE

If you like scary movies, and if you've ever imagined what it would be like to experience the zombie apocalypse yourself, then this is the race for you.

A zombie run is typically a 5K/3.1-mile race, often organized as an obstacle course. You can register either as a human, trying to get to the finish line without having your flag taken by a zombie, or you can be a "chaser"—a zombie runner who tries to take a runner's life by stealing their flag.

If this already sounds scary, wait for the kicker: Zombie races have professional makeup artists to make the zombies seem more lifelike (or dead-like?). Zombie runners are also instructed in how to stumble and crawl for maximum effect, and how to work together in packs in assigned "feasting zones" to corner runners. Costumes are encouraged, and races are offered not just in the daytime, but also at night.

If all of this sounds too intense for you, don't worry; the goal is still to have fun. There is a code of rules, and on-site referees who make sure that no zombie gets too aggressive. (Website: https://zombiefunrun.com/)

NOTES

. . . .

. . . .

. . . .

. . . .

● RUN A ZOMBIE RACE Date:...............................

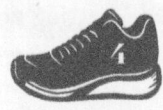

RUN A BEER RACE

Here's another racing challenge that will test your stomach as much as your legs. The idea is to run or walk 3 or 5K while partaking in 5 drink stops. If that wasn't enough of a test, the course also includes five obstacles, which range from traversing an inflatable obstacle course to jumping over hay bales.

It might not be for everyone, but for those who are willing to take up the challenge, this is the one of the quickest—if not easiest—ways to check off another item on your list. (Website: https://5kbeerchallenge.co.uk/)

NOTES

....
....
....
....
....
....
....
....
....
....
....
....
....
....
....
....

● **RUN A BEER RACE** Date: ....

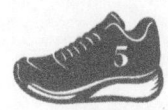

RUN A MUD RUN/ OBSTACLE COURSE RACE

If you're looking for something completely different to shake up your running, this is for you. Preconceptions about distance and time get thrown out the window when a racecourse includes wading through a mud pit, climbing walls, and crawling under wires. Be prepared to get very dirty, and to love it. There are many such races across the U.K.; a good place to start could be the Tough Mudder race series (website: www.toughmudder.co.uk).

NOTES

● **RUN A MUD RUN / OBSTACLE COURSE RACE** Date: . . . .

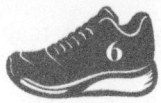

TACKLE THE EMPIRE STATE BUILDING RUN-UP

Most races take you a set distance on land. This one doesn't go far—just 1,050 feet, which is about one fifth of a mile. But the catch is that it's almost entirely straight up.

This is the first and most famous tower race, first run in 1978. It's a sprint up 86 flights of stairs, comprised of 1,576 steps, to the observation deck of one of the most iconic skyscrapers in the world. Most of the 500 racers will take less than 15 minutes to complete the event, with the fastest competitors completing the climb in about ten minutes. (The record is 9:33, set by Paul Crake in 2003.)

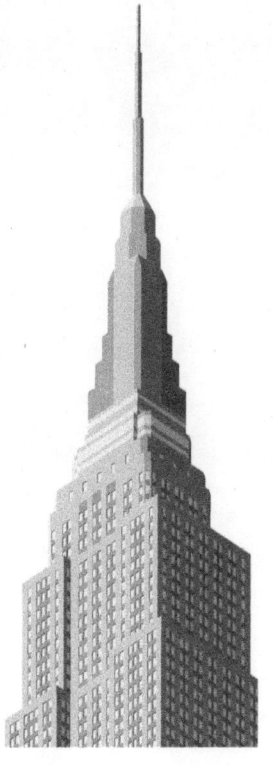

The race starts in the building's lobby, as waves of runners sprint to the stairwell to begin their climb. You can expect to heat up during the climb, which makes the sudden exit onto the outdoor observatory near the finish line a bit shocking, since the race is held in October, when the weather can get chilly, especially at that height.

Racers then proceed into the gift shop and take the elevator back down to the ground level, a return journey that will now take less than a minute to complete.

There will be no crowds to cheer you during this race, no bands playing on the course, and no aid stations. But you will likely get more bragging per step taken than any other race you'll ever enter. (Website: www.esbnyc.com)

NOTES

● **TACKLE THE EMPIRE STATE BUILDING RUN-UP** Date: . . . .

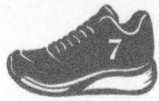

RUN IN FANCY DRESS

"Serious" runners may sneer at it, but there's something special about running in a costume. The joy comes less from your own experience, and more from the joy you create among your fellow runners and spectators along the course. Dinosaurs, monsters, superheroes, celebrities—there's room for all of them. Some races even encourage costumes, and give awards for the best outfits. (See, for example, the Bay to Breakers and the Marathon des Châteaux du Médoc, mentioned previously.) And in case you were thinking that runners who choose to race in costume must all be slow, there are speed records for various categories of race costumes.

When deciding on your own costume, keep in mind the length of the race and the weather conditions. A costume that might be fine to wear for a 5K could become a disaster in a marathon. But the point of trying this at least once in your life is to stop taking this all so seriously and have some fun. After all, it's just running.

NOTES

....
....
....
....
....
....
....

● RUN IN FANCY DRESS Date: ....

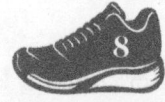

AIM TO FINISH LAST IN A RACE

In every race there is only one winner. Less considered is that there is also only one last-place finisher. While no one gives much thought to who is in the back of a pack of racers, being absolutely last is somehow more worthy of recognition. Some races even give out awards to the last-place finisher. And that's how it should be, since even the very last person to finish was still audacious enough to start a race, which puts them ahead of all the thousands of people who didn't even try. Spectators know this, since they usually cheer as loudly for the last few participants as they do for the winners. For those who worry they might be last, this should come as a pleasant surprise.

Many racers do not have a choice but to be at the back of the pack, but even if you are a middle-of-the-pack runner or faster, you should experience what it is like to be in the back. The camaraderie and support you find back there will make you love this sport all the more.

NOTES

....
....
....
....
....
....
....
....
....
....
....
....
....
....

● **AIM TO FINISH LAST IN A RACE** Date: ....

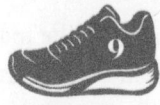

START A RACE IN LAST PLACE

It wasn't intentional. I was late getting to the start line for the Los Angeles Marathon—shame on me for not checking street closings before the race—so after a sprint from a cab to the start line, I discovered all the runners had already crossed the start line and gotten underway. But this was a chip race, so all I needed to do was cross the start line, and my own race would begin.

I thought I would be running the whole race angry, but I quickly realized I was in unique position. By starting last, I had let all the race participants surge ahead and spread out, and now I could do my sheepdog imitation and run after them, with the goal of passing as many as possible before clearing the finish line.

It was a different kind of challenge, and a different kind of experience—one that every runner should try at least once.

NOTES

■ START A RACE IN LAST PLACE Date: ....

DO THE ROCKY RUN CHALLENGE

If you're a fan of the *Rocky* movie franchise, or of Philadelphia, or of taking up a new kind of challenge, this is the event for you. Taking place in early November, this event consists of a 5K and a 10-mile race. You can run either, or—and here's the intriguing part—both! The 5K comes first, followed very shortly by the 10-mile race. The total distance raced equals a half marathon, but of course it's not exactly the same experience, since you'll be doing two races, likely with different pace goals and strategies, interrupted by a break of a half hour or so.

But for many participants, the real draw is the Rocky theme. Runners start and finish in front of the Philadelphia Museum of Art, in view of the Rocky statue that commemorates the famous stair run scene in the first *Rocky* movie. Continuing the theme, the participant shirts and finisher medals sport images of Rocky and his opponents, and, of course, choruses from the movies can be heard all along the course. Many runners like to race in costume, wearing Rocky's iconic red, white, and blue boxing shorts, and even red boxing gloves.

The course itself is beautiful. From the museum start, all racers head north for an out-and-back run along the Schuylkill River, past the boathouses in Fairmount Park. Ten-mile race participants continue on and race up a big hill, referred to by the race organizers as "Mount Drago," after the gargantuan boxer Ivan Drago portrayed by Dolph Lundgren in *Rocky IV*. The only thing missing is a run up the stairs at the finish. Though unfortunate, that's understandably not part of the race, presumably for safety and security reasons.

The finisher medals deserve special recognition. Participants compete for four different medals in one morning of racing: the 5K and 10 miler finisher medals, the Italian Stallion finisher medal for participants who complete both races, and the prestigious Mount Drago finisher medal for the first 100 male and female runners to conquer that hill. But it's not just the quantity of finisher hardware that should get your attention, it's the design of the medals themselves. Each of the four classes is distinct, and all are big, heavy, and incredibly elaborate. Imagine something like the centerpiece of a heavyweight boxing championship belt. They really need to be seen to be believed. You may need to bring additional luggage to Philadelphia just to get one home. (Website: https://rockyrun.com)

NOTES

● DO THE ROCKY RUN CHALLENGE Date:.........................

CHAPTER 9

6 Race Collections You Need to Have

- Abbott World Marathon Majors *(page 168)*
- 50 States Marathon Club *(page 171)*
- Seven Continents Club *(page 173)*
- Race the Poles *(page 175)*
- Country Check-Off List *(page 176)*
- Armed Forces Race Challenge *(page 178)*

Races often become like potato chips—it's hard to stop after just one. It's easy to see why that's so. Crossing a finish line is often the one completely positive event we have in our lives. Some people will come back to the same race year after year, building up a streak of race completions.

Others, however, look to run in related races. Whether grouped by geography, distance, or type, these races provide runners with an elevated sense of accomplishment, as well as a great excuse to travel around the country and the world.

Some of these collections are formally recognized by running organizations that honor runners who have completed the series. Others are informal groupings of races or runs that share certain characteristics. You can also come up with your own collections as well. I've known people who, for example, aimed to run every marathon held in Pennsylvania.

Grouping your races or runs in this way will not itself change your running, since each run is its own event. Indeed, you might be able to double dip in your bucket list achievements if your run is both a standalone event and a collection member. That's not cheating; that's just being smart and organized. Remember, too, that you are the one who makes the rules about your bucket list, so if you say double-dipping is allowed, then so it is.

The whole point of the bucket list, after all, is to identify running experiences that will motivate and inspire you and provide memories to last a lifetime. The bucket list described in this book is itself the ultimate run collection. But every runner should consider adding these running achievements to their list of lifetime accomplishments.

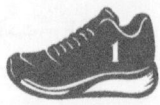

ABBOTT WORLD MARATHON MAJORS

Many sports have organized into championship series, with the best athletes in the world competing in events around the globe to determine who is the best in the sport. Golf and tennis, for example, have their series of Opens.

This had never been the case in running. Athletes and their coaches would decide on their race season, and certain races were known to draw the world's best runners because they offered big cash prizes and featured fast courses, but there was no system in place to determine an overall champion.

That changed in 2006 with the creation of the World Marathon Majors (WMM) (now Abbott World Marathon Majors). It established a point-based system that linked six of the world's biggest, highest-profile marathons into a two-year race series. These marathon host cities were Boston, Berlin, New York, London, Tokyo, and Chicago. Each of these races deserve to be on any runner's bucket list. You might even have been wondering why I hadn't mentioned them earlier. Well, here they are now.

Elite marathoners earn points in each event by placing within the top five finishers in each race. Fifth place earns one point, and the totals ascend through first place, which earns 25 points. To be eligible, an athlete has to compete in at least one of the qualifying races in each calendar year of the two-year series.

The pot of gold at the end of this rainbow totals over one million dollars in prize money, divided among the top five men and women runners and wheelchair athletes. As expected, the list of series winners reads like a who's who of the world's best marathoners.

The WMM has been a big boost to the sport, providing additional incentives and support for a sport that has not traditionally been very lucrative for its top performers.

Most importantly for us, however, the WMM is not just for elite athletes. Since 2016, any runner can aim to complete the race series and earn the prestigious Six Star finisher's medal. There is no time limit in which participants can complete their six-race odyssey, and there is no minimum finish-time for each race. As long as your time appears in the official race results, the WMM will credit you with finishing that race.

To participate in the WMM, runners need to create a portal on the organization website and then upload race finishes. If you've run any of the WMM marathons before the race series was created, you can still get credit for completing those events by submitting screenshots of your result or finisher's certificate along with proof of ID. When a runner completes the race series, they can receive a finisher's certificate, the Six-Star medal, and a place in the website's Hall of Fame.

The popularity of the WMM program has led to its expansion. In 2024, the TCS Sydney Marathon was added as a seventh event, and the Sanlam Cape Town (South Africa) Marathon and the Shanghai Marathon have been chosen as candidates for future inclusion. But striving runners don't have to be worried about having the goal move farther out of reach; completion of the original six marathons still results in recognition of having completed the WMM challenge, with completion of the TCS Sydney Marathon (and any future additions) qualifying participants for further medals and recognition.

Ultimately, the WMM's goal appears to be more than encouraging participation in these marquis events; it's to create a community of runners. On the WMM website you will find information about the Global Run Club, offering virtual training and racing challenges throughout the year, as well as a podcast and a magazine. (Website: www.worldmarathonmajors.com)

NOTES

....
....
....
....
....
....
....
....
....
....
....
....

● ABBOTT WORLD MARATHON MAJORS   Date: ....

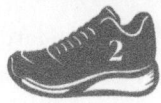

50 STATES MARATHON CLUB

This goal often sneaks up on runners. It begins simply enough, with one marathon finish followed by another. You might read or hear about an especially interesting marathon not too far away or organize a getaway vacation that includes a marathon. Before you know it, you realize you've managed to run marathons in six or seven or twelve different states, and then the thought occurs to you: Wouldn't it be a great achievement to run at least one marathon in every state?

Indeed it would. It would take planning, because while some states, like Pennsylvania and California, offer many different marathons, other states host only a few. But with some careful scheduling, you can make this happen.

If this goal appeals to you, then you are not alone. There is a club organized especially for runners working toward—or having achieved—this milestone. According to its website, the 50 States Marathon Club has more than 5,000 members, spread across all 50 states and 22 countries, who have run a combined total of

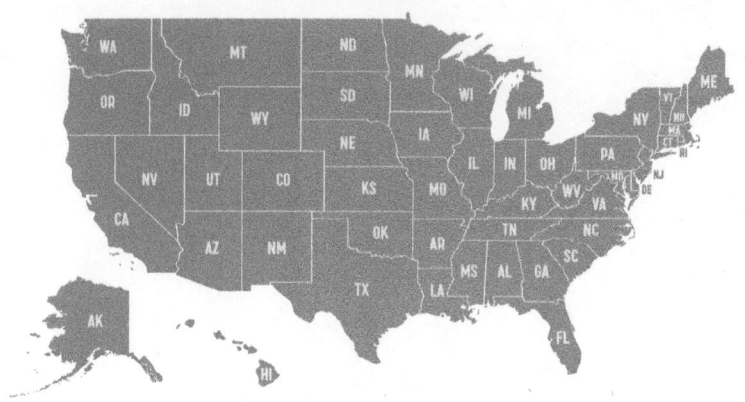

more than 383,000 marathons. Standard membership in the club is available to any runner who has completed marathons in at least 10 states, with full membership available to those who have completed marathons in all 50 states.

Perks of membership include discounts for club members at participating marathons, and regional club gatherings. Best of all, when you've collected marathons in all 50 states and submitted the necessary documentation to the club, you are listed on their Finisher rolls, and you will receive a beautiful 50-State Finisher award. For many runners, this award will be the culmination of a decade or more of hard work, and it will be their proudest accomplishment. (Website: www.50statesmarathonclub.com)

NOTES

● 50 STATES MARATHON CLUB Date:..........................

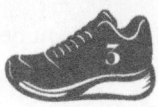

SEVEN CONTINENTS CLUB

This is a category that can challenge your financial fitness as much as your cardiovascular strength. It can start easily enough, with a marathon in North America and another in South America. Then the stakes get higher, with marathons in Europe, Asia, and Africa. Australia/New Zealand can be logistically difficult but is also manageable. You'll burn through all of your credit-card miles and more, but this can all be done. But then things get very tricky with the final stop: Antarctica.

Nailing the southernmost continent used to be a pipe dream for runners, but in 1995 the folks at Marathon Tours & Travel decided to take up the challenge and organized the first Antarctic Ice Marathon, for the ultimate in running bragging rights. Participation in this race is limited to approximately 360 runners, and those slots sell out quickly, so checking this one off your to-do list might take years of patient waiting. The trip itself entails signing up for a two-week excursion, starting with a flight first to Buenos Aires, and then continuing on to Tierra del Fuego at the tip of South America. From there, runners board a ship for a three-day cruise through the Drake Passage and down to the Antarctic Archipelago. From there they board an inflatable landing craft and land on King George Island, where the marathon will take place among scientific bases and glaciers. As one trip leader put it, by the time you leave Antarctica, the marathon won't even be among your top memories.

Recognizing that many of its customers were aiming to complete the seven-continents challenge, Marathon Tours & Travel also created the Seven Continents Club, facilitating entry into races and handling all the logistics. All you need to do is train and have your credit card ready. (Website: www.marathontours.com) In light of the great demand for these events, it was natural that competition would spring up. Case in point: the 7 Marathons Club. As of the writing of this book, that exclusive club boasted of having 479 members, including 359 men and 120 women. (Website: www.7marathonsclub.com)

But as the television commercial used to say, "Wait! There's more!" For those who want to push their bodies—and bank accounts—to the limit, there's the Great World Race, seven marathons on seven continents in seven days—and it *starts* in Antarctica! The logistics alone can be mind-boggling, but the physical challenge is real and formidable: approximately 184 miles within one week, across many time zones, in a wide variety of weather and terrain. Even for the most adventurous among us, this is a hard event to wrap our heads around. (Website: www.thegreatworldrace.com)

NOTES

....
....
....
....

● SEVEN CONTINENTS CLUB Date:.............................

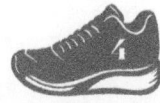

RACE THE POLES

As an additional challenge to the Seven Continents Club—after all, you would have already nailed the South Pole—or as an alternative, there is the Polar Club.

The premise is simple: two poles, two races. But you would be hard-pressed to find two marathons that will challenge you more than these two. We've discussed the Antarctic Marathon, and for greater authenticity you can run even closer to the true South Pole in the Antarctic Ice Marathon (website: www.icemarathon.com). But compared to racing at the North Pole, those races might be a piece of cake. Racing the world's northernmost marathon requires more elaborate transportation arrangements, as participants are landed on the polar icecap. But don't imagine that you have to suffer every step of the way; participation in the North Pole Marathon—billed as "The World's Coolest Marathon"—includes a luxury cruise as part of the adventure. But get ready for some sticker shock; notching the ultimate in running bragging rights won't come cheap. (Website: www.npmarathon.com)

NOTES

● **RACE THE POLES** Date: ....

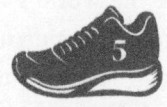

COUNTRY CHECK-OFF LIST

There are currently 195 nations in the world. I am keeping a running tally (pun fully intended) of all the different countries where I've been lucky enough to race. For me, the point of this isn't to just tick off more races in more places; it's that a road race—and especially a marathon—often represents the best way to experience a new place. Think of the race as a tour on closed city streets, fully supported with drink, snacks, and porta-johns, usually past the most scenic and historic sights a city or region has to offer. For many of us, there's no better way to see a new place. After the race, you can go back and explore the highlights at your leisure.

Having this goal can also make family vacation planning easier. Instead of insisting on specific races you want to travel to, you can solicit dream destinations from your family or friends and then look online for races there. The date of the race might limit your options, but if your goal is simply to race where you've never been before, you should have plenty of choices.

Taking this one step farther, you can encourage your family and friends to look up races where they want to travel, and present it to you that way. They might find this gives them far more control of vacation plans than they'd ever imagined having.

A great place to begin your search is at Marathon Guide (www.marathonguide.com). There, you can look up races throughout the U.S. and around the world by calendar date or location. The race descriptions include links to the official race websites, as well as reviews submitted by past race participants. Other useful sites include Running in the USA (www.runningintheusa.com) and World Athletics (www.worldathletics.org).

NOTES

. . . .

. . . .

. . . .

. . . .

● COUNTRY CHECK-OFF LIST Date:..............................

ARMED FORCES RACE CHALLENGE

This collection of races was decades in the making. First came the Marine Corps Marathon, traditionally held on the last Sunday of October. Established in 1976 as a recruitment tool, it became immensely popular, growing over the years to be the fifth largest race in the U.S. Starting and finishing at the iconic United States Marine Corps War Memorial (the "Iwo Jima" memorial) just outside Arlington Cemetery in Northern Virginia, this race tours the nation's capital, museums, and monuments on its way to the finish line. (Website: www.marinemarathon.com)

Over the years, the other services created races as well: The Army Ten-Miler came out in 1985. Taking place in early October, it is now the second largest race of that distance in the U.S.,[17] covering some of the same territory in Washington, D.C., as the Marine Corps Marathon. (Website: www.armytenmiler.com)

The Air Force Marathon came next. It was organized in 1997 in Dayton, Ohio, the home of the Wright Brothers' bicycle shop—the business they owned before taking up the dream of powered flight. Taking place on the third Saturday in September, the marathon brings participants onto Wright-Patterson Air Force Base, passing historic aircraft on the way to the finish line. (Website: www.usafmarathon.com)

The youngest of the set is the Coast Guard Marathon, created in 2022 and taking place every spring in historic Elizabeth City, New Jersey. The race flows along the city riverfront, passing through the Coast Guard Base and past World War II airship hangars, before finishing downtown. (Website: www.coastguardmarathon.com)

Recognizing that the total could be greater than the sum of its parts, these races came together to form the Armed Forces Series Challenge. You begin by going to any of the race websites and registering your intent to complete the challenge. You will need to register for each race individually. You need to register for the challenge before you can start collecting races, so you can't get retroactive credit for races that you've run in the past, but there is no time limit to completing your challenge. After you've crossed the five finish lines, you will receive the Armed Forces Series Challenge medal, and you can cross another item off of your list.

---

17 Top honors go to Philadelphia's Broad Street Run.

NOTES

....
....
....
....
....
....
....
....
....
....
....
....
....
....
....
....
....
....

● **ARMED FORCES RACE CHALLENGE** Date: ....

CHAPTER 10

8 Ways to Give Back

- Be a Race Volunteer *(page 182)*
- Race for a Charity *(page 185)*
- Be a Mentor *(page 188)*
- Be a Pacer *(page 190)*
- Be a Blind-Runner Guide *(page 193)*
- Be a Plogger *(page 195)*
- Thank the Volunteers and Police on the Racecourse *(page 197)*
- Cheer! *(page 199)*

"If I am not for myself, who will be for me? If I am only for myself, what am I?"

—Rabbi Hillel, philosopher and religious leader, 110 BC

As runners, we are naturally focused on our own individual experiences. We monitor our training, plan our race schedule, and track our performances down to the second. There's nothing wrong with that, but if that's all we do, then we're missing out on some of the best parts of being a member of this running community.

By moving outside of our own running and becoming involved with others, we get a chance to share our experiences as runners, and to support their efforts—to their benefit, but also to our own, because it gives us an opportunity to define who we are.

Remember: Every act of selflessness is a tribute to those people who helped us along our own journey—nameless people along a racecourse, or close friends who gave support when we needed it. Pass it on.

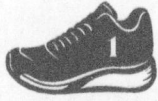

BE A RACE VOLUNTEER

We have all benefited from their work, and no race could exist without them. They hand out our race numbers and T-shirts at the pre-race expos, direct us on the racecourse, give us water and sports drinks at the aid stations, cheer us when we tire, and drape medals around our necks at the finish line. They are the volunteers who selflessly give their time and energy to everything from the small, local 5K to the mega-huge marathon.

Every runner should appreciate them, and every runner should try, at least once, to be in their shoes. Forego running a race and volunteer instead. It's not much of a sacrifice. Perhaps you're coming back from an injury, or you've already run your goal race for the season. In either of those cases, you wouldn't be running this race anyway, so get out there and be of service to the rest of the running community.

As described, there are myriad jobs that need to be done, and you can usually choose which one appeals to you. Perhaps you enjoy feeling the excitement at the expo or the starting line, or you like to be a cheerleader on the course. Or perhaps, like me, you like to be at the finish line, helping the walking wounded and sharing in the celebration of a job well done.

As a finish-line volunteer, you can learn a lot about the different kinds of runners who participate in races. There are the elite runners, who often seem to be in a world of their own. Then there are the strivers, who push themselves as hard as they can to get a breakthrough performance. These runners rarely seem to be aware of volunteers and often seem too deeply buried in their own struggle to thank the helpers around them.

Then there are the mid-pack and back-of-the-pack runners. These are a different breed entirely. They care about their race, but they are also usually just happy to be there, participating. They thank the volunteers for the cups extended to them, for the directions they give, and the medals they hand out. They are usually the happiest of all the participants out there.

I volunteer at races to give something back to the running community, after having been a recipient of their support so many other times. But I also volunteer to remind myself of why I run, and of what kind of runner I want to be.

Most races have a page on their official website on which you can sign up to be a volunteer. Once you do so, you will receive an email giving you specific instructions about where and when to show up for work. There will be a volunteer organizer on site who can answer questions you might have and take care of problems that might come up. You'll get to meet other volunteers, and you'll be given a volunteer T-shirt. For bigger races, you might also be given a volunteer jacket.

Don't be surprised if you end up enjoying your work, and if volunteering at races becomes a regular activity on your calendar.

NOTES

● BE A RACE VOLUNTEER Date: ....

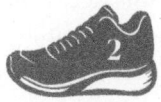

RACE FOR A CHARITY

Road races have traditionally had strong ties to charities. Many are organized by running clubs, which are themselves nonprofit organizations that rely on the races for sustaining funds. But beyond that purpose, many races have designated other nonprofit organizations to be beneficiaries of part of the participant registration fee. Ranging from supporting the homeless, to feeding the hungry, to fighting cancer or Alzheimer's disease, road races have raised many millions of dollars to do good in their communities and beyond.

All that is to be applauded, but we can do better: We can use our racing to conduct our own charity fundraising, whether by funneling donations through a race or working directly with a charity. However you do it, you may find that running for a cause adds meaning to your efforts, since it shifts the race from being only about you, to being about something bigger. It can also leave you feeling grateful to be healthy enough to race while many others cannot, due to illness or disability.

There are many worthy causes out there to choose from. One that I personally feel strongly about is the St. Jude Children's Research Hospital. Founded in 1962 by the entertainer Danny Thomas, it funds research of childhood cancer and turns laboratory breakthroughs into life-saving treatments, free of charge, to children in the U.S. and around the world.

St. Jude has established a strong runner-fundraising program through which it offers a wide variety of opportunities to the running community to get involved. They host the St. Jude Memphis Marathon Weekend in Tennessee, which features the marathon, a half-marathon, a 10K, and a 5K. Runners can also choose from a number of partner races, for which St. Jude will provide entries and online support for your fundraising efforts. Among the events offered are all of the races within the Abbott World Marathon Majors race challenge (see Chapter Nine). (Website: www.stjude.org/get-involved/fitness-fundraisers/run.html) With a little planning, you can mark several items off you bucket list by running a single race, all while trying to make the world just a little bit better.

NOTES

....
....
....

■ **RACE FOR A CHARITY** Date: ....

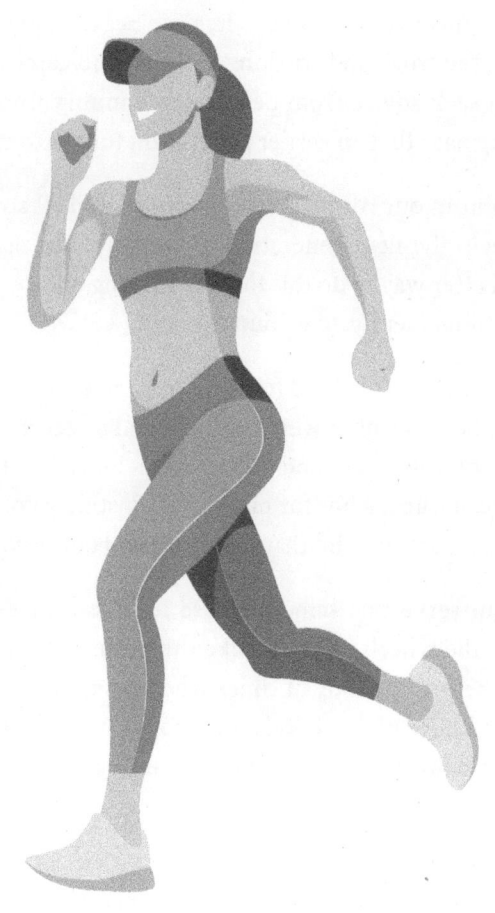

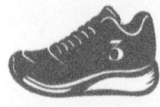

BE A MENTOR

In 1624, almost exactly 400 years ago, the poet and cleric John Donne delivered a sermon in which he told parishioners, "No man is an island, entire of itself; every man is a piece of the Continent, a part of the main."[18] His observation is as true now as it was then, and always will be: Like it or not, we are all interconnected.

For runners, this is easy to see. When we began running, we all made use of the work and wisdom of those who came before us, whether we seek advice from people at a running store or train on a running path that an earlier generation fought to create.

At some point in our running careers, we should all strive to inspire and help the next generation of runners. For many of us, there is no better way to do this than by making one-on-one contact as a running mentor to a young person.

As we get older, it's often hard for us to remember what it was like to be young. So many of us were confused and insecure as we tried to find out who we were and where we belonged in the world. Running became an anchor for many of us, instilling confidence, a work ethic, and a viewpoint that helped us find our way.

Running can serve this same purpose for the next generation. Let's grease the wheels a bit to make their journey easier, just as others had helped us along at times when we needed support. If you already know of some kids who could use mentoring, you can offer to help them out simply by talking with them about

---

18 www.dictionary.com/browse/no-man-is-an-island

their running, or inviting them to join you and your friends for an easy run.[19]

For many people, it's better from a logistical and liability standpoint to offer hands-on support to a formal, established youth development sports program. Whether organized as an after-school program at your neighborhood school, or by a nonprofit organization, these programs are always eager to make use of volunteers. Indeed, that is the only way they can operate.

Contact one and find out how you can help. Your support might range from handling team equipment, like snacks and water, to running with the group, to connecting with an individual athlete for more engaged direct support.

There is no right or wrong level of volunteering; do whatever you feel comfortable with, to the extent that you feel comfortable with volunteering. Like drops in the ocean, it all adds up. And remember, too, what a volunteer mentor once told me: You may never see the fruits of your work, but rest assured you are providing help to a young person that will change their lives, even if they don't realize it for years.

To find mentoring and youth development volunteering opportunities, contact your local running club, recreation center, school, running store, or England Athletics, who also offer training courses (https://www.englandathletics.org/). Be prepared to go through a screening process before you can begin.

---

19 It's crucial to emphasize that the run will be easy, and then to make sure that it truly is. Beginning runners often seem to think that every other runner will be faster than they are; they don't know, as we do, that some 80 percent of our running is in the easy zone. Once they see that running with a group won't be as hard and embarrassing for them as they'd feared, they are well on their way to becoming lifetime runners.

NOTES

....
....
....
....
....
....
....
....
....
....
....
....
....
....
....
....
....

● **BE A MENTOR** Date: ....

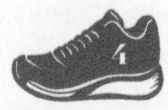

BE A PACER

You've probably seen them at races, and maybe you've even made use of their services. Pacers are the runners you see holding aloft a balloon or a banner on a stick, leading a pack of runners within the field of racers. On that balloon or banner is a number, which represents the finishing time that the runner is committed to finishing the race. Looking around at the starting line, you'll see balloons both ahead of you and behind. These are held by other runners, lined up to lead groups across a spectrum of speeds.

Those runners are pacers, and they have been officially tasked by the race organizer with providing a moving signpost to runners to help them achieve their race goals. They will set the pace so that participants don't have to worry about their speed. Pacers can usually offer guidance about the course—when hills are coming up, and where aid stations and porta-potties can be found on the course—as well as training and racing advice based on their deep experience.

To be a pacer yourself, you will have to be an experienced runner with a proven track record of running faster than the pace you will be expected to hold. For a marathon, this could be a finish that's 20 to 30 minutes faster than the goal time you will be assigned to. The pacer is expected to finish the race within a minute of the promised time. This can be a greater challenge than simply running the race. As a participant, you may expect to simply run as fast as you can, but being a pacer is a bit like throwing a dart across the city and hitting the bull's-eye.

Hitting your finish time is not your only challenge. You are also expected to hold even splits (i.e., maintain a consistent pace) along the course. On a hilly course, that may require you to focus on holding an even-effort level (i.e., a consistent level of energy), knowing that the slower runs uphill will be balanced by faster ones downhill.

If all of this gets you nervous, remember that no pacer is expected to lead a group by themselves. Two or more pacers are assigned to each time group, which ensures that if a pacer runs into trouble—and anything can happen to anyone on race day—they will have a backup ready to take over.

With all of these challenges, you may decide that pacing engages you more than simply running your own race.

To become a pacer, contact a race you are interested in pacing and ask for their pace team coordinator. The bigger the race, the more likely they are to have pacers. These days, almost all big or even midsize marathons are expected to provide pacers. They will want to know your training and racing background and may even ask you to "audition" at an upcoming race.

Your local running club may also have a pacer program, organized independently or in collaboration with a race. If you are already a member, it may be easy to get involved.

Finally, you may opt against being a formal pacer and simply offer to help your friends with their race. Whatever you choose to do, you can be assured that as a pacer, you will have a race experience unlike any other you've had before.

NOTES

....
....
....
....
....
....

● BE A PACER Date: ....

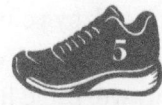

BE A BLIND-RUNNER GUIDE

Many of us take our vision for granted and never consider how very different our lives would be if we were visually impaired. It's almost impossible for many of us to consider how we could keep running if we lost our vision. Fortunately, there are organizations to help visually impaired runners of all ages to continue to train and race, and all they need is a volunteer like you to work with these exceptional athletes.

Visually impaired runners range from those who have some limitations, but who can still make out images, to those who are completely blind. They all rely on guides to run outdoors safely.

The most important tool used by running guides is the verbal cue. Guides call out any change in the upcoming path and call out a countdown. For example, a guide may say, "Curb in 3 … 2 … 1." They also call out any turns and upcoming obstacles. The rule is: "If in doubt, call it out."

Volunteers run side by side with their runner and often hold a tether to help guide the runner. They may also use touch cues and elbow leads. In races, guides may be needed to help with registration and review a race's particular rules for visually impaired runners.

Guides and support runners usually are first required to undergo background checks and complete training, and then will be paired with an athlete to help them achieve one or more of their possible goals—whether it is to conduct regular training runs, simply complete a race, or run as a competitive athlete.

This might seem a bit overwhelming, but as a blind-runner guide you will not be expected to work by yourself with the athlete; you will probably be part of a team. In that way you can manage your volunteer time around your work and life schedule, training and racing goals, and even, if necessary, your injury recovery periods.

Trust is obviously a big component of the guide-runner experience, so you, as the guide, and the runner will need to talk beforehand about boundaries and expectations. This trust helps build a relationship between the guide and the runner, and it is that relationship, and the running achievements you will together create, that is the most rewarding part of this volunteer experience.

There are many organizations that will train you and connect you with visually impaired athletes: England Athletics (https://www.englandathletics.org) and British Blind Sport (https://britishblindsport.org.uk/).

NOTES

● BE A BLIND-RUNNER GUIDE Date:..............................

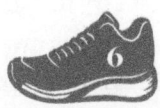

BE A PLOGGER

Runners see more of the streets than most people. We move slower than cars and cover more territory than pedestrians. Along the way, we often see a lot of trash. Bottles and cans, and wrappers and bags. On occasion, if I see some trash within reach while I'm out on a run, I'll grab it on the go and drop it off into the next garbage can. I feel pretty good about doing that.

In Sweden, they took my little effort to a whole new level, creating the activity of *plogging*. The term is a mash-up of *plocka upp*

(Swedish for "pick up"), and *jogga*, which—you guessed it—means jogging. Its origin is credited to Erik Ahlstrom, who started picking up trash on his runs through Stockholm in 2016.

The media seized on this and started spreading the word, and soon it became a global phenomenon. Today, there are an estimated 2,000,000 people who plog daily in 100 countries worldwide. There's now even a plogging organization that holds a World Plogging Championship. Don't ask me how that works, but you can check it out for yourself at Plogging.org (www.plogging.org).

As an activity, plogging can augment your running by adding more movements to your routine, such as squatting and reaching, which will enhance your fitness. Plus, of course, you will be doing your part to beautify your city and clean up the planet.

When plogging, there are certain safety tips you should keep in mind. Bring a moderately sized reusable bag and wear gloves. Consider bringing a grabber tool, and do not attempt to pick up anything that might be potentially dangerous, like medical waste or hazardous materials. Don't try to carry more than you can reasonably handle on your run, and be aware of any cars, bikes, and pedestrians around you. Be careful as you bend over—I prefer to protect my back by squatting more than bending.

NOTES

....
....
....
....
....
....

● BE A PLOGGER Date:......................................

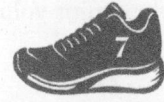

THANK THE VOLUNTEERS AND POLICE ON THE RACECOURSE

It's easy to take them for granted, because we are usually so focused on maintaining our pace and hitting our goals, or simply making it to the finish line, but without the volunteers on the course who hand out water and direct us and cheer us on, and the police who monitor street crossings and hold up traffic for us, no race would be possible.

You know this is true if you have already checked off the first bucket list item in this chapter and volunteered at a race. This is the flip side of that item, the place where you can now show some love for the people who give their time and energy to help make the race happen, for nothing more than just a "Volunteer" race shirt.

You might think that thanking volunteers on the course is such an obvious thing to do that we would not even need to make this a bucket list item, but most runners are so engaged in their own race that they don't give volunteers a second thought. But when you thank a volunteer, an interesting thing often happens—other runners will thank them, too. It's as if we've woken them up from their dazed state, and they realize they should show appreciation as well. So, when you thank a volunteer, you're not just showing them your appreciation, you're also prompting other runners to do the same.

I like to let as many volunteers as possible know that I see them and appreciate them. I'll try to make eye contact and address them directly. When it's a volunteer cheering me on, I like to respond in kind: When they say, "You're looking great!" I smile and answer back, "You, too!" The senior volunteers usually laugh appreciatively.

I also like to thank the police who block the intersections for us on race day. Even though they might be getting paid for their service, they still deserve our expressed gratitude.

If you are a parent, this is an especially important example to set for your kids. There's never a time when expressing gratitude is a bad idea, and that's a great lesson for our kids to learn.

NOTES

....

....

....

....

....

....
....
....
....
....
....
....
....
....

● **THANK THE VOLUNTEERS AND POLICE ON THE RACECOURSE** Date: ....

CHEER!

There are times when you won't be racing. Perhaps you've got a different race on your calendar, or you're recovering from an injury. Maybe you simply were unlucky and didn't get into the race, or you simply did not feel like racing. Whatever the reason, you don't have to be an official race volunteer to be supportive on the course. Just go out and cheer the runners as they stream past.

People who know me can tell you that I might have a tendency to overthink some things. That might be true—I'll have to think about it. But I have devoted some time pondering where is the best place to cheer on runners. As a spectator, it's no doubt the finish line, where you can see the winners cross the tape and urge on all the rest behind them to give it their all. But when I think about where it is on the course that I've appreciated cheering the most, I come up with two spots.

First, pick the emptiest spot on the course. If there's an intersection that seems to draw hundreds of cheering supporters, you don't really need to add your voice to the din. But if there's an out of the way bit of road, far from the cafes and shopping areas that might be an appealing convenience for spectators, go there. That's where your voice will be heard the loudest.

I'm reminded of the Marine Corps Marathon course in Washington, D.C., back in the late 1980s. There was a stretch of race around Hains Point, an isthmus that juts into the Potomac River. That area was always a dead zone. Worse, it was around mile 21, where runners can hit the dreaded Wall, that moment when their energy has run out and their legs feel like lead. But back then, appearing like an unlikely angel, there was an older man standing beside the open trunk of an old car, out of which he blasted the iconic theme song from the movie *Rocky*. It was magical, and it gave more than one runner the energy and will to go on.

The second place you can line up to cheer is the two-thirds mark of the race. This is the spot that, regardless of the race distance or the runner, can be the most challenging. It's where racers begin

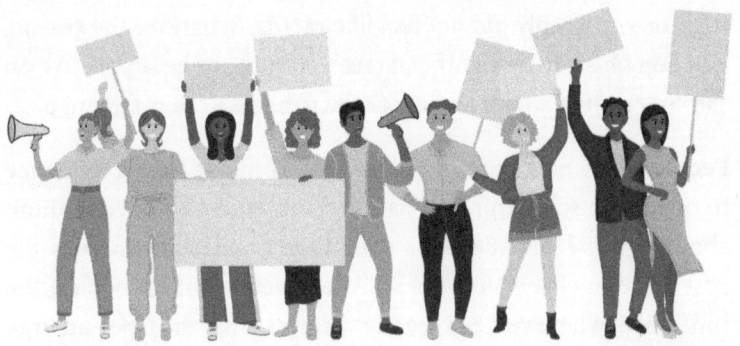

to feel the effects of the pace they've set for their race, whether they're trying to run a fast 5K or pushing themselves through a marathon. It's where doubts can begin to creep in, and they begin to wonder whether they'll be able to make it to the finish. This is where you're needed most. If there is no one else there to cheer, try to become a loud, one-person crowd, and if there are others already cheering, add your voice to the cheers of the others.

You can also plan to be a migrating cheerleading squad. If you have a bicycle, you can find it easy to zip around the course to cheer runners at different points.

Wherever you are on the course, try to make the cheering as personal as possible. Call out the person's race number or cheer them by name if they've got that written on their shirt or race bib. Offer useful information, like how far the next aid station might be, or the next mile marker.

On a side note, don't fail to take your own well-being into account. Bring food and drink, and dress appropriately, especially if it's cold outside. The runners are working up a sweat, but you'll just be standing there shedding body heat, possibly for hours. But most of all, have fun.

NOTES

....
....
....
....
....
....
....
....

● **CHEER!** Date: ....

CHAPTER 11

4 Ways to Be a Racing Fan

- See the Millrose Games in New York City *(page 204)*
- Watch the Commonwealth Games *(page 206)*
- See the USA Track and Field Championships *(page 207)*
- See the Olympic Games *(page 209)*

Almost everyone can run, but only a very few can do so at an elite level. Those special few seem almost otherworldly to the rest of us, and their performances can verge on the heroic. But they also struggle and battle through injuries and doubt, just like the rest of us. Being runners ourselves gives us special insight and understanding of their accomplishments, and seeing them perform can be fascinating and inspirational.

Can you be a runner without ever watching a track meet? Of course, but you would be missing out on an interesting part of our sport. Pick a major meet, find out something about the athletes who will be competing, and immerse yourself in the event. You won't regret it.

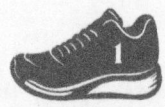

SEE THE MILLROSE GAMES IN NEW YORK CITY

In 1908, the employees of the John Wanamaker Department Store organized the Millrose Athletic Association as a recreational club and initiated an athletic competition they called the Millrose Games. They held their event in the Park Avenue Armory, in New York City, but it proved so popular that by 1914 they were forced to move to the more spacious Madison Square Garden. The games were held there annually, through a depression and two world wars, and several relocations of the Garden, until 2011, when it moved to the Fort Washington Armory, in Washington Heights. For many people, the highlight of the games is the Wanamaker Mile. Originating as a mile-and-a-half race, it was shortened to the mile distance in 1929 and has remained so ever since. Held on a temporary wooden track in the old Garden, the Wanamaker Mile has, during its long history, attracted the greatest runners in the sport. Originally held as a Friday night event, the games are now an all-day affair held on a Saturday in February. Arrive early and watch all of the track and field events. But do not miss the Wanamaker Mile. (Website: www.Millrosegames.org)

NOTES

■ SEE THE MILLROSE GAMES IN
NEW YORK CITY Date: ....

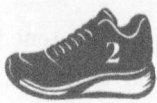

WATCH THE COMMONWEALTH GAMES

The Commonwealth Games are a multi-sport event held every four years for athletes from the Commonwealth of Nations. At present there are 74 countries from across the globe that are eligible to compete in the Games, including Kenya, Singapore, Barbados, and New Zealand. The event is hosted in a different city each time, with the 2026 Games hosted in Glasgow, Scotland.

Also called the Friendly Games due to its mission to unite nations through celebrating sport and promoting friendship and fair play rather than pure competitiveness, the Commonwealth Games were first held in 1930 in Hamilton, Canada. Back then it was called the British Empire Games and hosted only 11 countries competing in six sports: athletics, boxing, lawn bowls, rowing, swimming and diving, and wrestling. The next games are a far larger affair with a 10-sport programme, including six fully integrated Para Sports.

The Youth Games are also held every four years, with the 2027 Games in Malta. Both events are a brilliant showcase for international sport and a real celebration of sportsmanship. (Website: www.commonwealthsport.com)

NOTES

○ **WATCH THE COMMONWEALTH GAMES** Date: ....

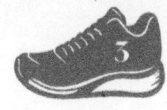

SEE THE USA TRACK AND FIELD CHAMPIONSHIPS

This competition traditionally takes place over four days in early July. It will determine the U.S.'s best athletes from high school through the professional ranks, with winners to represent the U.S. at the World Athletics Championships held later in the summer.

The USA Track and Field Championships traditionally take place at the University of Oregon in Eugene, on the historic Hayward Field, known affectionately as TrackTown USA. This gives you a chance to mark two items off your bucket list, since running on

Hayward Field is also something that all runners should aspire to. (See Chapter Six.)

Plan your spectator weekend by looking up the list of events, which will take place both indoors and outdoors, on the track and on roads and even trails, in categories ranging from youth through open, para, and masters participants. (Website: www.usatf.org/events)

NOTES

- **SEE THE USA TRACK AND FIELD CHAMPIONSHIPS** Date:

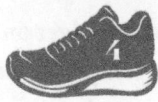

SEE THE OLYMPIC GAMES

This is a trickier item to mark off your list, since it is held only once every four years, and because travel and related expenses can create many logistical and financial hurdles to overcome.

Still, if you ever have the opportunity to see the Games, I recommend you do so. There is no prize money involved, but for many athletes, success in the Games is the pinnacle of their careers. For runners from Africa in particular, the cultural pressure to participate and perform well in the Games can be immense, and top athletes are expected to be on the national team, regardless of their professional plans. If they do well, they become national heroes. Here, you will see the world's greatest athletes competing head-to-head on the track and on the roads. There is nothing else quite like it in the world.

There are several ways to approach being a spectator at the Games. You can take a scattershot approach and buy cheaper tickets to the opening rounds for an array of events in order to get a better overall view of the Games. Or you can go all-in on your favorite events, blowing your budget on the gold medal round for just your favorite events, going for quality of competition over quantity. And remember, too, that you don't have to have a paid ticket to be in the Olympic Stadium to enjoy the marathon; you can track the race for free as it winds through the host city's streets.

Including attendance at an Olympic Games on your bucket list might be a difficult decision for you, and not just because of the financial and planning challenges. I understand that the Games are objectionable to a number of people because of the history of corruption among its officials, its negative impact on the environment, its escalating cost to host cities, and its commercialism, as well as its use by some host countries to suppress protest and push poor and indigenous people out of sight. Claims of cost are routinely underestimated, and claims of long-term economic benefit are wildly exaggerated. All of this has all been well-documented.[20]

Some of the Games themselves have made some attempts to correct some of these abuses, with some limited success. Whether the Games are inherently flawed or just need to be more closely monitored and controlled is for you to decide. The Games have always reflected the contradictions and challenges that our world has faced, and while they have not always been a force for good, at their best, they have been a stage for some of history's greatest and most inspiring athletic achievements. For that reason alone they are worth considering.

As I write this book, the next scheduled Games will be held in Los Angeles, California, from July 14 through 30, 2028, with the Paralympic Games to follow from August 15 through 27. You can sign up now for ticket updates at www.LA28.org.

---

[20] See, for example, *Power Games: A Political History of the Olympics*, by Jules Boykoff (Verso Press, 2016).

NOTES

....
....
....
....
....
....
....
....
....
....
....
....
....
....
....
....
....

● **SEE THE OLYMPIC GAMES** Date:..............................

CHAPTER 12

9 Great Runs You Need to Experience

- Run the Diamond Head Summit Trail in Oahu, Hawaii *(page 213)*
- Run the Cheddar Gorge Trail *(page 215)*
- Run the Walls of Pisa in Italy *(page 216)*
- Run on a Beach *(page 218)*
- Run a Timed Mile *(page 219)*
- Run Rim2Rim2Rim in the Grand Canyon *(page 222)*
- Run the Chesapeake & Ohio Canal Towpath *(page 226)*
- Run the Appalachian Trail *(page 228)*
- Run the Inca Trail in Peru *(page 230)*

The greatest runs I've ever had did not require me to register, pay a participation fee, or pin on a race number. They just asked me to get out there for a journey on an unforgettable route.

While you may find running on your favorite neighborhood trail to be completely satisfying, there are certain routes around the world that are unique and especially beautiful and should absolutely not be missed.

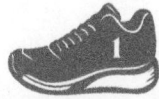

RUN THE DIAMOND HEAD SUMMIT TRAIL IN OAHU, HAWAII

Built in 1908 as part of a coastal defense system, this is a 1.6-mile round-trip path that leads to the top of Diamond Head volcano.

It begins innocently enough as a paved trail but quickly turns to dirt and includes stair climbing at its steepest sections as it rises 560 feet from the crater floor to the summit. There, visitors will find historic bunkers and a navigational lighthouse and breathtaking views of Honolulu.

The trail can be strenuous, especially for running, and heat can be a factor. Waikiki is only about three miles from the trail, so if you're staying in a hotel there, you can plan to run to the park, ascend, and run back for a total run of about eight miles.[21] (Website: www.dlnr.hawaii.gov/dsp/hiking/oahu/diamond-head-summit-trail)

---

21 Honolulu is about six miles from the park, making an out-and-back run the equivalent of a challenging half-marathon.

NOTES

● **RUN THE DIAMOND HEAD SUMMIT TRAIL IN OAHU, HAWAII** Date:...............................

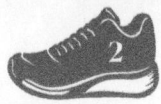

RUN THE CHEDDAR GORGE TRAIL

As well as being the home of the popular cheese, Cheddar Gorge is England's largest gorge at almost 400 feet (122m) deep and 3 miles (4.8K) long. Running this trail gives you the opportunity to soak up the surroundings of one of the UK's most spectacular sights.

Although the route is only 4 miles (6K), there's plenty to encounter along the way, including several stiles and kissing gates, and some pretty steep climbs. There'll also be a chance to spot some wildlife and historical points of interest along the way, including peregrine falcons, Feral Soay sheep and the famous Cheddar Gorge itself, which is thought to have first formed around a million years ago, during the ice age.

NOTES

● RUN THE CHEDDAR
GORGE TRAIL Date:............................

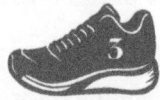

RUN THE WALLS OF PISA IN ITALY

If you travel to see the fabled Leaning Tower, you'll discover that Pisa is more than just the fourteenth-century tower; it's an ancient walled city in Tuscany near the mouth of the Arno River, home to a beautiful cathedral.

The defensive walls of Pisa are among the oldest such walls in Italy. Construction took place between AD 1154 and 1346. The Walls have undergone restoration, and a 3K stretch of these ramparts is now open to the public.

For runners, the walls of Pisa are an irresistible attraction. But be warned: There seems to be disagreement among the guards atop the walls as to whether you are allowed to run. Tourists typically walk the path, but when I ran it, I found that some guards cheered me on as I ran past, while others cautioned me to only walk. So, it seems running is fine, unless you're told otherwise. I'll caution you to always follow the directions of the guards, and be courteous to them, but you should aim to check this one off your list if at all possible.

Whether you can run on all or part of the walls, or choose simply to walk, you should try to go when there are fewer tourists, either early in the morning or later in the day, near dinnertime.

NOTES

● **RUN THE WALLS OF PISA IN ITALY** Date: . . . .

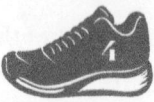

RUN ON A BEACH

There are more great beaches in the world than we have time to identify, but whichever you pick, give beach running a try. Running on the sand is a unique experience, and if you've never done it, it can be much more challenging than you might think. That's because the shifting ground changes the dynamics of your push-off, altering your biomechanics and putting more stress on your Achilles tendons. The sand can also act as an abrasive if you run barefoot, or even if sand gets into your shoes.

With all of this in mind, aim to run near to the water's edge, where the waterlogged sand is packed tighter. You should also keep your beach runs short until your body adapts to the differences. To get the best of both worlds, aim for beaches that also have runnable sidewalks or paved trails adjacent. The National Trust have a handy list of coastal runs on their website if you are in need of inspiration: https://www.nationaltrust.org.uk/visit/outdoor-activities/best-places-for-coastal-running. But wherever you go, the salty sea air and sun should leave you refreshed and looking forward to your next run.

NOTES

● **RUN ON A BEACH** Date:..................................

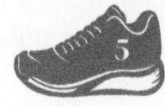

RUN A TIMED MILE

It's true—this run is not about experiencing a particular place, and it's not about beautiful scenery, although you can choose a beautiful location anywhere in the world to do this run. It's only and entirely about the run.

The mile was once the premier racing distance in the world, and the standard upon which runners measured their fitness.[22]

---

22   The metric system has replaced the English system of measurement over most of the world, and most international competitions have now replaced the mile with 1,600 meters as the standard race distance. Standing firmly in opposition is an organization whose mission is to return to the mile as the standard race distance in the U.S. and abroad. Visit Bring Back the Mile (www.bringbackthemile.com).

Indeed, breaking the four-minute barrier for the mile is widely considered to be one of the greatest athletic feats of the twentieth century. (See Chapter Six.)

Most endurance runners consider the mile to be simply one part of a longer—sometimes a *much* longer—run. We collect miles in training and racing the way some people might collect stamps and coins; they simply add up. But every runner should challenge themselves, at least once in their lifetime, to running a single timed mile as fast as they can.

To be done properly, you should use a standard track to ensure that the distance is accurate. Warm up thoroughly—there will be no time to warm up—and settle into a comfortable pace during your run, since it will be over so soon. If possible, see if a friend who is faster than you are would agree to be your pacesetter, running just slightly ahead of you to set a target and goal for your running. Set your timer—or better still, have a friend time you from trackside—and go!

If you've never raced a mile on the track before, you'll find it's much more than simply running four laps. Each of these circumnavigations feels different.

On the first lap, you'll feel strong and confident, because you are warmed up and excited, and no lactic acid has built up yet in your legs from the hard effort.

On the second lap, you're working hard, but you're probably still feeling quite fresh and strong as you settle into your pace.

The third lap, for my money, is the most challenging lap. You're now feeling the effects of those first two hard laps, as your legs feel heavier, and your breathing becomes more and more labored. You've come so far, but you've still so far to go; not just this lap, but another one after that. This is the moment when you have to grit your teeth and get tough, remind yourself that you only have a few minutes of running left, and that you can endure more suffering for just that short span of time.

Once you set out on the final lap, everything has changed again. You now can truly imagine being done; you have only two turns and two straightways until the finish line. As you get closer and closer to the end, you may find a last little bit of reserve that will enable you to suffer just a bit more and go faster. On that last straightway, you know you don't have to hold anything back, and you can run as fast as you possibly can.

When you fly across the finish line, you'll be gasping, but don't stop. If you're timing yourself, tap your watch quickly to capture your time, and slow down into an easy jog, and then into a walk, as you let your heart rate slow down and your breathing return to normal.

In all likelihood, this will have been the fastest pace you've ever run. Be proud of yourself. You've now got a measurement of your top speed, and it's something you can remember and cherish for the rest of your life. But don't be surprised if, shortly after you've cooled down and your legs feel good again, you begin to wonder if, maybe, with a little more training and speed-work, you can run even faster. And maybe you can.

NOTES

....
....
....
....
....
....
....
....
....
....
....

● RUN A TIMED MILE Date:...................................

RUN RIM2RIM2RIM IN THE GRAND CANYON

This is the legendary run that is on the bucket list of almost every runner I've ever met. It doesn't even require any explanation. A runner will just say "rim to rim to rim," and if you know, you know. Nothing more needs to be said.

It's a fairly straightforward course to run. You take the North Kaibab Trail on the north rim of the Grand Canyon, down through 11 layers of rock formation spanning two billion years of the Earth's history. On reaching the Colorado River and the Phantom Ranch lodge and campsite, you continue on the Bright

Angel Trail up to the south rim. The route is 24 miles—just under the 26.2 marathon length—making the roundtrip 48 miles. If you ran this on a flat road, the distance would qualify as an ultra-marathon and would be challenging. But this is no flat road. The descent is just over 14.3 miles, taking you down 6,000 feet, and the ascent will take you up 4,500 feet over the course of 9.6 miles. Then you turn around and do it again, in reverse. That's 21,000 feet in elevation change.

That would be hard enough on a nice day, but when considering a trip to the Grand Canyon, weather is always a factor. Conditions are often unpredictable, as the spring can bring snow and the summer, scorching midday heat. Deciding when to attempt the run forces you to face difficult choices. Do you try to avoid the heat by running in the transitional spring and fall seasons? But the days are shorter then, and you might find yourself in low light or darkness. So, do you decide to risk the heat and run in late June or early July, when you can enjoy the longest amount of daylight? Or do you compromise by doing one leg, and not the roundtrip? Or do one leg, spend an overnight on the opposite rim, and then complete the run on the next day?

Once you've decided how and when you want to run it, you have to decide on gear to bring. Tour companies offer a Rim2Rim guided hiking experience, or you can plan your own hiking adventure, but that's not what we're talking about here. This isn't a backpacking adventure; it's an epic run, and the rules are different.

I'm reminded of something I read years ago about the first successful transatlantic flight by Charles Lindbergh. He is said to have considered all of the failed attempts and concluded that by packing so much heavy emergency equipment, the pilots had set up conditions for failure. Lindbergh decided to forego all the emergency supplies and travel fast and light. If he failed, it would not be because he was traveling too heavy.

I don't know if that tale is true, but the principle applies to a Rim2Rim2Rim run. If you plan to backpack down and camp at Phantom Ranch, then you can afford to bring lots of supplies, but if you are going to run it as an ultra-marathon distance out and back, you should bring only what you must, and nothing more.

Your primary concerns on this adventure will be nutritional: You need to make certain you have enough fuel and liquids. A running pack with a large reservoir would be ideal; you can take sports drink powder to mix fluids on the go when you refill at the campground at Phantom Ranch and at the turnaround on the South Rim. You also need to take whatever energy bars or other foods have proven effective for you. Aim for high-calorie foods that pack a good energy punch for their weight.

Your clothing choices will be important as well. With weather subject to dramatic swings, you need to have many lightweight options that you can add or shed as needed. A thin shirt or singlet, a heavier long-sleeved shirt, a light waterproof jacket, and hat and gloves are a must. And this is a dirt trail, not a paved path, so you should consider using trail shoes and collapsible or folding hiking poles. Depending on what time of year you decide to tackle this run, a lighting system—whether a headlamp, hand-held flashlight, or both—could be necessary.

With so many moving parts involved, it would be a good idea to do a few trial runs with all of your equipment on a local trail before the big event. Practicing will reveal whether your plan works or needs improvement and will also boost your confidence for the upcoming challenge. The aim is to put as many risk factors in your favor as possible.

Most importantly, don't forget to take a moment (or twelve!) to stop and look around. You are on the run of a lifetime, on one of the most breathtaking trails in the world. Consider how lucky you are to be doing what you love in such an awesome place.

NOTES

....
....
....
....
....
....
....
....
....
....
....
....
....
....
....
....
....

● **RUN RIM2RIM2RIM IN THE GRAND CANYON** Date:................

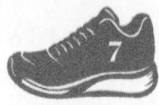

RUN THE CHESAPEAKE & OHIO CANAL TOWPATH

The history of this trail almost matches its beauty. Built between 1828 and 1850, the Chesapeake & Ohio Canal was intended to bring coal from western Maryland to Washington, D.C., which at that time had a thriving port. By the time the canal was finished, however, the Baltimore and Ohio Railroad was completed, and it took over much of the canal's business. Nevertheless, the C&O Canal continued to operate for nearly a century. In 1924, a flood caused major damage to the canal, and due to its decreasing profitability and the costs of repair, it was largely abandoned. In 1938, it was taken over by the U.S. government.

In 1954, a plan was proposed to turn the canal into an automobile highway, but Supreme Court Justice William O. Douglas thought that was a terrible idea. Justice Douglas had overcome the effects of polio by hiking as a young man near his hometown of Yakima, Washington, and he viewed the canal as a beautiful natural resource. He had taken to doing Sunday hikes along the canal towpath, which ran along the length of the canal, providing a path for mules to pull the canal barges.

Justice Douglas responded to the proposed plan with an editorial in the *Washington Post* in which he argued in favor of protecting the canal. He then organized a hike of the entire canal to gain publicity and support for his cause. Justice Douglas didn't make it the entire way, but his scheme paid off when the plan was withdrawn. The canal endured, but it was not until 1971 that the canal was designated a National Historical Park. Fittingly, it was officially dedicated to Justice Douglas.

The canal is 185 miles long. It is measured by short wooden mile markers and contains 74 locks and 11 aqueducts. Campgrounds can be found every 10 miles or so, and there are also cabins that can be reserved for a fee. And everywhere there are beautiful views of the Potomac River.

Along the way, the canal passes through the historic town of Harpers Ferry, where the abolitionist John Brown infamously led a raid on the federal armory located there on October 16, 1859, hoping to arm slaves for a rebellion he envisioned. John Brown and his men were captured after a standoff of several days, and later hanged, but the Civil War that he saw coming could not be so easily avoided.

At any given time, and especially on Sunday mornings, you can find individuals and packs of runners training on the canal, especially closer to its terminus in Washington, D.C. Cyclists ride the canal to the start in Cumberland, where they connect onto the Great Allegheny Passage trail, which takes them over the Eastern Continental Divide and into Pittsburgh, Pennsylvania.

The canal, then, can be whatever you need it to be. Do regular training runs, or have an epic multiday run-and-camp adventure. But get out there and enjoy this amazing resource. (Learn more about the Chesapeake & Ohio Canal National Park at www.nps.gov/choh/index.htm.)

NOTES

- RUN THE CHESAPEAKE & OHIO CANAL
  TOWPATH Date:..

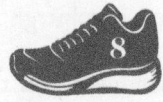

RUN THE APPALACHIAN TRAIL

This trail is epic in its length and audacious in its conception: a nearly 2,200-mile-long trail crossing through 14 states on the eastern United States seaboard, from Springer Mountain in Georgia to Mount Katahdin in Maine. The Appalachian Trail Conservancy, a nonprofit founded in 1925 to partner with the U.S. government to manage the trail, claims that it is the longest hiking (and running!) trail in the world.

First proposed in 1921 and completed in 1937, it was formerly designated the Appalachian National Scenic Trail, and is less formally known simply as "the A.T." It ranges in altitude from a low of 124 feet above sea level near Bear Mountain in New York state, to a high of 6,643 feet in the Great Smoky Mountains of North Carolina. It is home to the American black bear, as well as a number of venomous snake species.

Apparently, people just can't get enough of the A.T. It attracts over three million visitors annually, and among these are a strange breed called the "thru-hikers," who aim to hike the entire trail in a single season. The Appalachian Trail Conservancy estimates that over 3,000 visitors attempt thru-hikes each year, of which about a quarter succeed.

For dedicated trail runners, conquering the Appalachian Trail is the ultimate challenge—not by hiking, and not over the course of a season, but by running it in a single shot. Elite trail runners aim to post a Fastest Known Time, which uses GPS and other data to verify completion times.

The current Appalachian Trail Fastest Known Time record is held by Tara Dower. In 2024, at age 31, she completed the entire trail in 40 days, 18 hours, and 5 minutes, beating the previous record by an astounding 13 hours. To do so, she averaged 54 miles per day.

You may have no interest in running the entire A.T., whether all at once or in segments over the course of a season or many seasons. But at some point, every runner should get their trail shoes dirty on the A.T., even if only for a day. Plan your adventure online. (Website: www.appalachiantrail.org)

NOTES

● RUN THE APPALACHIAN TRAIL Date:..............................

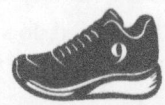

RUN THE INCA TRAIL IN PERU

For many people, this is the ultimate bucket list item. Because of its popularity, this trip might require the most planning. The Peruvian government has strictly limited access to the trail because of fears of erosion, and it closes the trail every February for conservation and maintenance work, so you will probably need to plan this well in advance of your target date.

Permits are required, and only 500 people are allowed on the trail daily, including guides and porters, so you will probably have to book your adventure through a guide service. But don't let these logistical challenges stop you—the adventure is well worth the effort.

Machu Picchu is a near-mythic stone sanctuary built by the Incan civilization in the fifteenth century, high in the Andes Mountains in southern Peru. Because the Incans did not have a written language, the actual purpose of this ancient city is not known, but archeologists believe it was built to be a royal residence and was occupied from 1420 to 1532. Home to as many as 750 residents, the mountain city is an architectural marvel, containing advanced drainage, water management systems, and terraced farming. The city was abandoned and soon became overgrown with jungle foliage, but it was not forgotten. For centuries, it existed as a legend and became a point of fascination for Western colonizers. In 1911, American historian and explorer Hiram Bingham III was led to the site by a Peruvian villager, and he organized major clearing and excavation of the site the following year, revealing the incredible ancient city that is so well-known today.

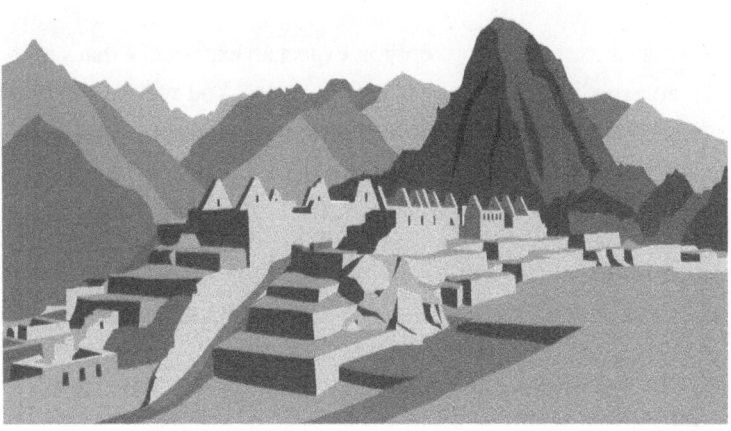

In 1981 Peru designated a 125-square-mile area surrounding Machu Picchu as a historic sanctuary, and in 1983 UNESCO designated it a World Heritage Site, calling it "a masterpiece of art, urbanism, architecture and engineering."[23]

The Inca Trail is a network of ancient roads that lead up to Machu Picchu. It contains moderately difficult stretches, but also easy descents. Along the way, visitors will have incredible views of cloud forests and alpine tundra, wildlife, and, of course, Incan ruins. The greatest challenge of the trail, however, is the altitude, which tops out at 13,779 feet above sea level, when the trail passes Dead Woman's Pass, named for a rock formation that resembles a reclining female.

A favorite of hikers, the Inca Trail can also be an incredible running experience. You can find a number of options to meet your adventure goals. If you are race-oriented, there is the Inca Marathon Vilcabamba-Machu Picchu Marathon and Half-Marathon, taking place in September (www.eriksadventures.com), or the Inca Marathon, taking place in May (ultrasignup.com).

If your goal is to experience trail running in a less formal race atmosphere, you can take a run tour of the Trail (for more information, visit Runcation Travel's website: www.runcation.org).

Whichever experience you opt for, expect an experience that's more like an expedition than a one-day adventure. You will visit various sites and learn about ancient Inca as well as modern Peruvian culture. On the trail, whether racing or trail running, expect a great deal of stair climbing, especially as you near Machu Picchu itself.

Preparation for this experience will need to be more extensive as well. As a coach, I'd recommend a stronger emphasis on strength

---

23 "Historic Sanctuary of Machu Picchu," UNESCO World Heritage Centre, UNESCO

over speed, incorporating lots of hills into your runs, and strength work into your training. In terms of gear, you would need to be prepared for a range of climates, so plan to pack a wide range of clothing, including lightweight rain gear. You will also be exposed to the possibility of altitude sickness, so you should consult with your doctor about taking medication with you.

However you intend to tackle this adventure, I would suggest that your goal should be to enjoy the experience, rather than to aim for a great running performance. If you want to run fast, sign up for a local race in your hometown. When you go to the Andes, don't be in a rush. Take your time and stop to smell the llamas. Well, maybe not literally. But you get the idea.

NOTES

● **RUN THE INCA TRAIL IN PERU** Date: ....

CHAPTER 13

6 Ways to Be Entertained as a Runner

- Listen to a Running Podcast *(page 235)*
- Create a Go-To Playlist of Running Songs *(page 238)*
- Memorize "To an Athlete Dying Young" *(page 241)*
- Visit the Running Statues *(page 243)*
- Read These Books *(page 246)*
- See These Movies *(page 251)*

Running is about movement—at whatever speed and for whatever distance you choose. But some running experiences aren't about movement at all. Instead, they touch us in different ways, making us laugh, think, wonder, or maybe even cry. Writers and film producers seem drawn to running and have produced work that tries to help us understand what it means to be a runner, and why such a simple act seems to matter to us so much.

Experience the items on this list, and then take the memory of that experience out with you on the roads, and spend a little time with it. You won't regret it.

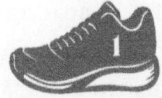

LISTEN TO A RUNNING PODCAST

Coaches talk about two types of training modes: associative and dissociative. The former involves staying mentally engaged in the act of running, focusing on how our body feels and anticipating the conditions that we're encountering. The latter involves distracting ourselves from the act of running so that time flies by. Associative running is more closely related to achieving high performance, while dissociative running is more closely related to recreational running. (For more on this, see Chapter Three.)

One type of running is not inherently better than the other, and it's common for runners to move seamlessly from one mode to the other, as our goals and moods dictate. When engaged in dissociative running, there are several different ways we can distract ourselves. We can listen to music—and we'll talk about that in the next section—or we can listen to running podcasts.

If we choose podcasts over music, we can pick a variety of them that can educate, inspire, and entertain us, providing not just a distraction from running, but a vehicle for enhancing our appreciation and understanding of our sport.

There are many running podcasts to choose from. The list of those that are available at any time are subject to change, and, of course, which ones are the best is a matter of opinion. You should ask your running friends for their recommendations, but in the meantime, here are some choices that are widely accepted as being among the best. Of course, you don't have to run while listening to these podcasts, but if you do, you might find that the miles fly by more easily.

The Rich Roll Podcast. Hosted by an ultra-marathoner and author, each podcast features special guests ranging from Boston Marathon winner Desiree Linden to actor Matthew McConaughey. Over the two hours of each podcast segment, Rich talks about many topics, including, of course, running.

Nobody Asked Us With Des & Kara. Hosted by champion professional runners Desiree Linden and Kara Goucher, this podcast gives you entertaining insights and information on the world of running.

Marathon Training Academy Podcast. Over a decade old, this podcast is the perfect site for tips on training and racing, hosted by coach Angie Spencer and her husband Trevor.

Doctors of Running Podcast. This is the show for people fascinated by the science of running. Doctors discuss such topics as running shoes and the physical and mental aspects of running, and also answer listeners' questions.

The Human Race. Even though this show was canceled, you can still access its 29 episodes, and it's well worth your time. Here you'll find inspirational and amazing stories.

Maybe Running Will Help? Hosted by elite runner Nicky Tamberrino, each episode is a conversation with an invited guest, ranging from the legendary Bart Yasso, to doctors, coaches, athletes, and even yours truly, to explore the physical, mental, and emotional aspects of running.

NOTES

● LISTEN TO A RUNNING PODCAST   Date: ....

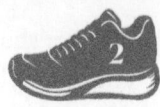

CREATE A GO-TO PLAYLIST OF RUNNING SONGS

For many runners, there is an inextricable bond between running and music. Perhaps it's because running itself is so rhythmic, or perhaps distance running gives us the time and space to enjoy a great song, or twenty. Or maybe it's because music helps distract and motivate us through our runs. Whether it's piped into our ears through headphones, or blasted out of speakers live or recorded on racecourses, running and music just seem to go together.

Your musical taste is your own, and there obviously is nothing right or wrong about what you listen to. A song with a strong beat that matches your target cadence seems like a good pick, but I've known runners who like to run to classical music.

I know there's a lot of new music out there to stream, but I still go old school when I run. There are certain songs that just seem to me to be perfect for running. I know that I'm biased, but I believe that every runner should start with these and then add to the list with their own favorites.

"Born to Run," by Bruce Springsteen. There is no more iconic running song in the world. From its opening chords through its anthemic chorus, the signature Springsteen song tells a story of hope and desire and the need to escape our limits to pursue our dreams. It's not specifically about running, but there's no better song to run to.

"Runnin' Down a Dream," by Tom Petty. The lyrics seem to capture how many of us feel about our running, and the catchy strumming in the chorus never fails to put a little more energy into my legs. This one is a keeper.

"Where Are We Runnin'?" by Lenny Kravitz. You could actually pick any one of Kravitz's big hits to run to, but this one seems especially appropriate for our focus. Enjoy the song and answer the rhetorical question for yourself.

"Hells Bells," by AC/DC. This song sneaks up on you, slowly building from its opening notes until it explodes on you like a tsunami of sound. You don't have to be a big AC/DC fan to appreciate the way this song can move you, although it helps.

"Stairway to Heaven," by Led Zeppelin. This is where I really show my age. A perennial pick for best rock song of all time in radio station countdowns through the 1970s and 80s, this song broke the mold for length and complexity for a rock song. It's also great to run to. I speed up every time I hear it. And at about eight minutes in length, you might even squeeze in a mile or more before it's over.

"Rhapsody in Blue," by George Gershwin. Surprised to see this work listed with those others? Don't be. This piece of music is like running itself, bringing us through different moods until it builds to a resounding climax. It was first performed at a daylong jazz concert in New York City on February 12, 1924. Some members of the audience, tired from hours of sitting through a largely uninspired concert, were leaving when the first strains of the song, a clarinet solo, rang through the hall. Those audience members froze in their steps and returned to their seats. At the end of the piece, the audience erupted in rapturous applause. Perhaps this piece of music will have the same effect on you, and on your running.

NOTES

....
....
....
....
....
....
....
....
....
....
....
....
....
....
....
....
....
....

● **CREATE A GO-TO PLAYLIST OF RUNNING SONGS** Date: ....

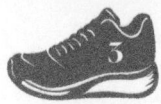

MEMORIZE "TO AN ATHLETE DYING YOUNG"

Running hasn't sent many poets into swoons of creativity, extolling the deeper virtues of our beloved sport. Perhaps that's why this poem stands out. Penned by the English romantic poet A. E. Houseman (1859–1936) and included in his collection *A Shropshire Lad*,[24] this poem reflects on the briefness of youth and glory through the lens of running. It may not spark a love of poetry in you, but at the least it will give you something to think about on your long runs and perhaps impress your running friends. Here it is, in its entirety:

To an Athlete Dying Young

The time you won your town the race
We chaired you through the market-place;
Man and boy stood cheering by,
And home we brought you shoulder-high.

Today, the road all runners come,
Shoulder-high we bring you home,
And set you at your threshold down,
Townsman of a stiller town.

Smart lad, to slip betimes away
From fields where glory does not stay,
And early though the laurel grows
It withers quicker than the rose.

---

24 First published in 1896.

Eyes the shady night has shut
Cannot see the record cut,
And silence sounds no worse than cheers
After earth has stopped the ears.

Now you will not swell the rout
Of lads that wore their honours out,
Runners whom renown outran
And the name died before the man.

So set, before its echoes fade,
The fleet foot on the sill of shade,
And hold to the low lintel up
The still-defended challenge-cup.

And round that early-laurelled head
Will flock to gaze the strengthless dead,
And find unwithered on its curls
The garland briefer than a girl's.

NOTES

● MEMORIZE "TO AN ATHLETE DYING YOUNG" Date:................

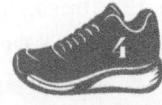

VISIT THE RUNNING STATUES

If public statues are a declaration of a community's values, then it should be no surprise that running statues can be found in cities across the globe. Here are the ones that no runner should miss.

JOHNNY KELLEY STATUE IN NEWTON, MASSACHUSETTS. If it can be said that one man can completely embody a race, then that man was Johnny Kelley, and the race was the Boston Marathon. In 1935 he won the race, but he was only getting started. He would go on to run the race 60 more times, ending his streak when he was 84. He would win the race again in 1945, and come in second place seven times, while finishing in the top ten on 19 other occasions.

In 1936 he was leading the race going into the final six miles when he was passed on a big hill in Newton. A spectating journalist named it the hill that broke Johnny Kelley's heart, known to hundreds of thousands of marathoners since as Heartbreak Hill.

After hanging up his running shoes, Kelley became the grand marshal of the race, riding in a convertible on race day on the course he loved so much. Before the race start, Kelley would stand on a stage before the thousands of participants in the runners' village who were waiting for the start of the race and serenade them with his signature song, *Young at Heart*. At that moment, there was nowhere else that a runner would want to be.

In 1993, a seven-foot-tall statue sculpted by artist Rich Muno was unveiled in Newton, on the marathon course, not far from the base of Heartbreak Hill. It depicts two runners holding hands as they breast the tape at the finish line: a 27-year-old Kelley winning the race in 1935, and an 84-year-old Kelley finishing his final Boston Marathon.[25] Appropriately, the statue is named "Young At Heart."

FRED LEBOW STATUE IN CENTRAL PARK, NEW YORK CITY. Founder of the New York City Marathon, and its longtime race director as president of the New York City Road Runners Club, Lebow changed the face of running and helped create the modern mega-marathon. After Lebow lost his long battle with brain cancer in 1994, this statue of him was dedicated at the finish line of that year's edition of his signature race in a ceremony attended by 23 former winners of the race.

The statue, created by Jesus Ygnacio Dominguez, depicts Lebow positioned at a race finish line, wearing a tracksuit and his signature race cap, checking the time on his wristwatch. The statue now stands nearby in Central Park at 90th Street and East Drive, keeping an eye on the runners streaming by. But on marathon race day, the statue, like its namesake, can be found once again standing near the finish line.

---

25 Johnny Kelley passed away on October 6, 2004, at the age of 97. His headstone reads, "Marathon Man."

DROMEAS (THE RUNNER) IN ATHENS, GREECE. Along the course of the Athens Marathon (see Chapter Six) is this work created by Costas Varotsos in 1988, moved to this site in 1994. It's made up of thousands of pieces of jagged glass stacked one atop the next, creating an unforgettable blurry image of a huge runner in motion. It is as close as we may come to seeing speed frozen in time.

PAAVO NURMI STATUE IN HELSINKI, FINLAND, AND LAUSANNE, SWITZERLAND. Cast in 1925 in bronze by the sculptor Wäinö Aaltonen, this statue depicts one of history's most accomplished runners in mid-stride. Named "the Flying Finn," Nurmi dominated running in the 1920s, setting 22 world records in middle-distance racing and winning one gold and three silver Olympic medals.

Nurmi posed for the statue, but it was designed not as a naturalistic portrayal, but as an idealistic monument to running. Nurmi is depicted in the nude, like a classical Greek figure, and is on his toes, running as if weightless. Two can be viewed at the front field of the Helsinki Olympic Stadium, and at the Olympic Museum Park of the International Olympic Committee in Lausanne, Switzerland.

NOTES

....
....
....
....
....
....
....

● **VISIT THE RUNNING STATUES** Date: ....

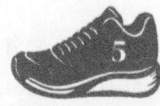

READ THESE BOOKS

The great Paavo Nurmi (just discussed) once said, "Mind is everything. Muscle—pieces of rubber. All that I am, I am because of my mind."[26]

Runners understand this. We spend hours out on the roads, trying to distract our minds, quiet our minds, work with our minds, and overcome our minds to achieve our goals. Maybe it's this internal struggle that makes running a good subject for writers, who put into words the experiences that all runners share in training and racing.

There are as many different types of books about running as there are, well, books. From training and racing guides to memoirs

---

26 www.brainyquote.com/quotes/paavo_nurmi_311931

and novels, running has served as a vehicle for us to explore our bodies and ourselves. There are many great books about running for you to explore out there, but at a minimum you need to read these.

The Loneliness of the Long-Distance Runner, **by Alan Sillitoe (W.H. Allen Ltd., 1959).** A short story in a collection bearing the same name, this is a story of an alienated young man who discovers running while serving time in a facility for juvenile delinquents. Through running, he discovers more about himself, and uses his running to rebel against the class system he feels has boxed him in. A prototype of the "runner as rebel" that we see in other works of fiction, such as *Once a Runner* (see below), and in real life (Steve Prefontaine, whom you will meet on page 252), this story was later made into a feature movie that is also worth your time.

Running & Being: The Total Experience, **by George Sheehan (Penguin Books, 1978).** This is a book that offers medical advice and practical tips on running, but also so much more. Sheehan's musings on running and life became the philosophical explanation of the sport, reflecting ourselves back to us with a clarity and grace that transcended running. When Sheehan, a cardiologist and elite master runner, wrote, "Run like a child," he was speaking about more than training or racing. He was advising us on how to live.

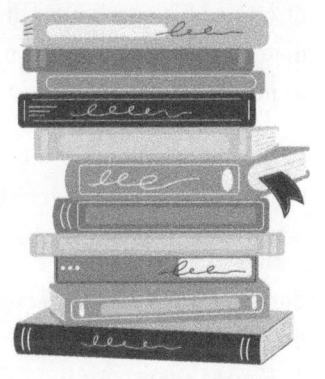

Once a Runner, **by John L. Parker, Jr. (Scribner Books, 2009).** First published in 1978, this novel quickly became a cult classic.

When it was out of print for a few years, copies were passed along hand-to-hand, sometimes in mimeographed form.

It is a semi-autobiographical story about one Quenton Cassidy, a collegiate miler at a Florida university, who pursues his dream of running a sub-four-minute mile as he negotiates the turbulent politics of the 1960s. After being expelled from school, he continues to run on his own, and gains the support of a former Olympic runner, who coaches him to a climactic race at the end, in which he hopes to purge his demons and achieve his potential against the best runner in the world. The best parts of this book focus on the mindset of a runner and the mental journey of an athlete struggling to achieve his potential. While few of us have the talent that Cassidy does, we can all relate to his struggles. For years, I kept returning during my runs to an image from the book: Cassidy's realization that the goal of training is to remove the outsole of his shoes, molecule by molecule. The description of one of his workouts—a seemingly endless repetition of 400-meter sprints that leaves him past the point of exhaustion—comes to mind during my hardest track workouts.

Parker later returned to Cassidy in a second novel, *Again to Carthage*. While it was a pleasure to reconnect with Cassidy and see where he was heading, there was nothing like the first meeting.

Born to Run: A Hidden Tribe, Superathletes, and the Greatest Race the World Has Never Seen, by Christopher McDougall (Alfred A. Knopf, 2009). An investigative nonfiction story about a secret trail race in the Copper Canyons of Mexico, this book is equal parts science, biography, and adventure tale. McDougall takes us into the world of evolutionary biology, introducing us to the scientists who are working to explain the genetic legacy we all carry that enables us to become long-distance runners. He also introduces us to a character known as *Caballo Blanco*, the White

Horse, a mythical runner who haunts the Copper Canyons of Mexico. McDougall manages to track him down, and he turns out to be a real flesh-and-blood American expat with the unlikely name Micah True, who is pursuing his own dream of the perfect solitary life.

We learn also of the Tarahumara, a tribe of indigenous people renowned for their distance-running excellence. Rounding out this unlikely cast of characters are ultra-marathon champions Scott Jurek and Jenn Shelton, and a runner known as Barefoot Ted.

These runners come together for the highlight of this book: a 50-mile challenge race through the Copper Canyons. McDougall plays Dante for us, narrating this descent into a kind of hell.

This book became a runaway bestseller, and it's not hard to see why. We come away from it wiser for the experience, understanding more about these athletes, the worlds they live in, and ourselves.

***The Perfect Mile: Three Athletes, One Goal, and Less Than Four Minutes To Achieve It*, by Neal Bascomb (Mariner Books, 2004).** Most of us know that, in 1954, Roger Bannister became the first man to run a sub-four-minute mile. (See Chapter Six.) What is less well known is the competition he had with two other runners, the American Wes Santee and the Australian John Landy, to be the first person to achieve that distinction, and their fierce competitions afterwards. This book is almost as thrilling to read as it must have been to watch them race.

***What I Talk About When I Talk About Running*, by Haruki Murakami (Knopf Publishing Group, 2008).** A memoir by the Japanese novelist who has run more than 20 marathons. You may relate to his reasons for running, and his description of the place it holds in his life: "For me, running is both exercise and metaphor."

Murakami recalls for us his time owning a jazz club, his decision to become a novelist, his training for the New York City Marathon, and his experience running the Athens Marathon.

The Terrible and Wonderful Reasons Why I Run Long Distances, by The Oatmeal (Matthew Inman) (Andrews McMeel Publishing, 2014). Not a deep, cerebral book, or a how-to guide, this is a funny, semi-serious and deeply relatable book about why it is we put on our running shoes and head out the door.

NOTES

● **READ THESE BOOKS** Date:

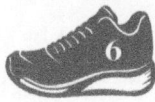

SEE THESE MOVIES

Running is not an armchair sport. It requires physical commitment to movement. Most runners don't even like to be indoors; they'd much rather be out on the roads or trails than indoors on a treadmill.

How strange it must seem, then, to see a bucket list category for runners that requires us to be indoors, probably sitting still (although no one would stop you from setting up a treadmill in front of your TV).

But this category isn't about becoming a stronger or better runner, or about running faster, or about avoiding injuries. It's about finding inspiration and being entertained. Each of the movies in this category will make you appreciate running in a different way, whether with a laugh, a tear, or a simple nod of appreciation. They will each stay with you after the screen goes dark and give you something to think about on the roads, and in your races.

Are these great movies? Some of them are, and some of them aren't, and we may disagree over which movie belongs in which category. But all of them are worth watching.

Saint Ralph **(2004).** It's 1954 at a Catholic school in Ontario, Canada, and student Ralph Walker is a troublemaker. After the headmaster puts Ralph on the cross-country team to take some of the resistance out of him, Ralph discovers that his mother has slipped into a coma. Ralph gets it in his head that if he can manage to win the Boston Marathon, God will grant his prayers and make his mother well again. After all, one miracle deserves another. His dedication to his dream is noticed by Father Hibbert, a former elite marathoner himself, who decides to help Ralph on his quixotic quest.

Clichéd, predictable, and even saccharine-sweet? Sure. But that doesn't mean it isn't fun. Give it a watch, and get inspired.

Chariots of Fire **(1981).** This film's theme song by Vangelis became the background music for a generation of runners. The movie itself tells the true story of two British runners pursuing their dream of competing in the 1924 Paris Olympics: Eric Liddell, a devout Christian born to Scottish missionaries who runs to bring glory to God, and Harold Abrahams, a Jewish runner who is striving to overcome antisemitism and class bias.

This film won Oscars for Best Picture and Best Score, but the scene that seared itself onto our memories is of the team of athletes running on the beach, full of strength and energy and life. There may be no finer image than that of the pure joy of running.

Without Limits **(1998).** Steve Prefontaine was an icon of running in the early 1970s. A breakout track star, he ran for Coach Bill Bowerman at the University of Oregon, winning 119 of 151 outdoor track races he competed in, including six NCAA titles. He set 15 American records at distances from two miles to the 10K/6.2 miles, and he represented the U.S. in the 5K at the 1972 Olympic Games, running a risky and courageous race, but ultimately failing to win a medal.

It wasn't just his running prowess that he was famous for, however. It was *how* he ran. Pre, as he was known, shunned conventional strategy and insisted on running at the front of a race pack, pushing the pace, instead of sitting back in the pack and going for the win in a late sprint. For Prefontaine, it was a matter of philosophy. "To give anything less than your best is to sacrifice the gift," he famously said. "I am going to work so that it's a pure guts race at the end, and if it is, I am the only one who can win it."[27]

This attitude—of seeing a race as a test of will, and raising it up to the level of art—won a huge following, but Prefontaine's career and life came to a tragic end in a fatal car accident when he was just 24. But the legend of Pre lives on.

There are not just one but three movies about Pre—a documentary, entitled *Fire on the Track: The Steve Prefontaine Story* (1995), and two biopics, *Prefontaine* (1997) and *Without Limits* (1998). For my money, the best of the lot is *Without Limits*, starring Billy Crudup as Pre, and Donald Sutherland as a cranky coach Bill Bowerman. The ending will break your heart, but the film will make you want to lace up your running shoes and race out the door.

Brittany Runs a Marathon (2019). A charming comedy about a woman with emotional and physical challenges who decides to turn her life around by training for and running the New York City Marathon. Funny and inspiring, it's based on a true story— one that many viewers will be able to relate to.

Run Fatboy Run (2007). A rom-com directed by David Schwimmer and starring Simon Pegg as Dennis, a bridegroom who leaves his pregnant wife, Libby, at the altar, and then tries to win her back. Since being jilted, Libby has gotten together with nice guy Hank Azaria, and now, five years later, she is running a marathon for charity. Dennis decides that if he can run the race also, he might be able to win her back, even though it takes place in just three weeks. This movie won't change your life, but it will give you some laughs, and some lessons on what *not* to do.

---

27 www.brainyquote.com/authors/steve-prefontaine-quotes

***Running Brave* (1983).** Based on the true story of Native American runner Billy Mills, it's the story of Mills's struggle to overcome racial stereotypes on his way to an unlikely victory in the 10K at the 1964 Tokyo Olympics. We know the ending before it begins, but that's true for every roller-coaster ride as well. Just buckle in and enjoy the journey, especially the beautifully filmed concluding Olympic race.

***Forrest Gump* (1994).** This movie won a basketful of Oscars over 30 years ago and spawned a bunch of catchphrases into our culture. None was more pervasive than the exhortation "Run, Forrest, run!"

Not specifically a running movie at all, *Forrest Gump* was memorable for many of us for its sequence of Gump as a long-distance runner, trekking across the country, driven on by an urge that he can neither understand nor articulate. The earnestness of his running turns him into a kind of running guru in the film, as he attracts a band of runners who follow him, hoping for a glimmer of some kind of enlightenment.

They won't find any, and we're not sure that Gump really does either, but watching him run definitely resonates with many of the runners in the audience. I'm betting it will resonate with you as well.

***Run Lola Run* (1998).** A conceptually interesting and beautifully filmed high-energy action movie, this is a story about Lola's efforts to save her boyfriend, Manni, a bagman who is about to get killed for bungling a cash drop-off to his criminal boss. Manni has lost the money and desperately calls Lola for help. She's got 20 minutes to get there to make things right. She races out the door and sprints to Manni to fix things, avoiding—or not avoiding—obstacles on the way.

Lola's sprint to Manni is as exciting as any running sequence ever filmed, but what makes this film especially interesting and different is that rather than giving us a single version of the story, the director rewinds Lola's run and gives her multiple chances to get it right, changing the dynamics a bit every time. You'll root for Lola from the edge of your seat as she sprints through her crazy race.

The Hustler **(1961).** I was torn about whether to include this film on our bucket list, since it isn't really about running at all—even less so than the previous recommendations. In fact, it doesn't contain a single image of anyone running. But still, this black-and-white classic movie has influenced my running, and it might do the same for you.

Paul Newman stars as a small-time pool hustler, "Fast" Eddie Felson, and Jackie Gleason joins him as Minnesota Fats. Rounding out the stellar cast are George C. Scott as Felson's ruthless manager, and Piper Laurie as Felson's troubled love interest.

This is a movie about pool players and the people around them, but it is really much more: It's a movie about character, and the loss and suffering that must be endured in building it. Those are themes that many runners can deeply relate to.

Possible spoiler alert: There's a scene early in the movie where Felson has challenged Minnesota Fats to a game of pool, which inevitably turns into an all-night endurance contest. The hours—and, for Felson, alcohol—set in and take their toll on the players. At one point, Fats goes to the wash basin. He splashes some water on his face, dries himself off with a hand-towel, and then turns to Felson with renewed vigor and says brightly, "Okay, Eddie, let's shoot some pool," as if they were just starting to play.

This image has been a powerful one for me late in my marathons and ultra-marathons, and I've used Fats's challenge as a mantra to reset my own focus. "C'mon," I say to myself when I feel especially tired, "let's shoot some pool." And it works.

NOTES

⬤ **SEE THESE MOVIES** Date:..

CHAPTER 14

Moving Forward

Now that you've reached the end of this book, you might be experiencing varied emotions. Hopefully, you feel inspired by what you've just read, and eager to check these items off your list. I've felt that way myself as I've been writing it, wondering whether I should return to those runs and races I've already done, and commit to doing those I've listed but not yet experienced for myself.

There's also the possibility you might be feeling somewhat indignant that the races and runs you thought would surely be here were left out. Or maybe annoyed that I've included some items you think didn't deserve to be here. That's fine. To paraphrase The Dude from the 1998 Coen Brothers movie *The Big Lebowski*, this book is just, like, my opinion, man.

But really, think of this book not as a comprehensive and complete list of running events, but as the start of the conversation. Ignore the items that don't resonate with you. There will be no penalty for that. Do you have items that didn't make it into this book? Come up with as many as you can and then write them down in the margins, or on the inside of the covers.

Then share them—with me, and with others. But only if you want to. Your bucket list, and your accomplishments, are your own, and if you need to keep them private, that is entirely your prerogative. You have no obligation to share them, any more than you have to share your personal dreams. But if you do decide to share them, you may inspire others, and in our sport, there is perhaps no greater achievement than that.

Remember: A bucket has a finite space, but a bucket list can be endless. As long as we have breath in us and energy to run, there are adventures to be had. The journey isn't over until we say it is.

Acknowledgments

Having a book published is always a privilege. I am forever grateful to the whole team at VeloPress for their faith and support, and particularly to my editor, Kierra Sondereker, and her endless supply of enthusiasm.

I am also deeply grateful to all of my readers. Thanks for giving my books a chance. Being a contributing member of our running community has meant the world to me. Thanks especially to those readers who have contacted me with their thoughts, comments, and stories. I always enjoy hearing from you. See you on the roads!

About the Author

Jeff Horowitz is a certified running, cycling, and triathlon coach and a personal trainer who has run more than 200 marathons and ultra-marathons across six continents. Formerly an attorney, he quit law to pursue his passion for endurance sports. He currently teaches running and strength training at George Washington University and works with athletes from ages 14 through 80. Horowitz is the author of *Quick Strength for Runners, Smart Marathon Training: How to Run Your Best Without Running Yourself Ragged, My First 100 Marathons: 2,620 Miles with an Obsessive Runner, Ageless Strength: Strong and Fit for a Lifetime,* and *Think Like a Runner.*

Taking a book from manuscript to market is a team effort. This book was carefully created by:
Publisher: Jo Morrell
Commissioning Editor: Katie Forsythe
Editorial Assistant: Sarah Ramnath-Budhram
Creative Director: Mel Four
Project Editor: Rimsha Falak
Production Controller: Sarah Parry
Sales: Lucy Helliwell and Natasha Photiou
Marketing & Publicity: Matilda Ngute and Karen Baker